change the way you

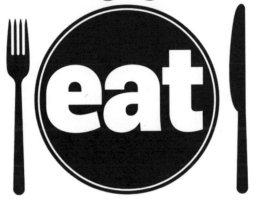

Leanne Cooper is an author, educator, nutrition consultant and advisor. A registered nutritionist, she is the founder and director of Cadence Health (Australia, NZ, UK), dedicated to enhancing community health through food coaching, quality online training courses, books, and free resources and information. Leanne initially trained to be a childhood psychologist but gradually shifted her focus to health. *Change the Way You Eat* combines both areas of expertise — psychology and nutrition — as Leanne delivers her message that by understanding the psychology of food we can take back control of our health.

change the way you

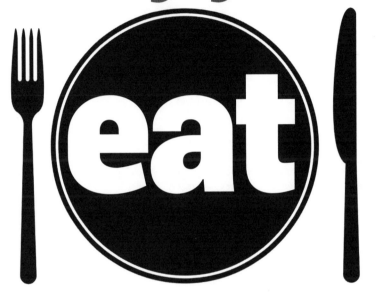

The psychology of food

LEANNE COOPER

BA (Psych/Ed), GCertHumNutr

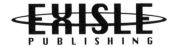

EXISLE
PUBLISHING

First published 2014

Exisle Publishing Pty Ltd
'Moonrising', Narone Creek Road, Wollombi, NSW 2325, Australia
P.O. Box 60–490, Titirangi, Auckland 0642, New Zealand
www.exislepublishing.com

A CiP record for this book is available from the National Library
of Australia

ISBN 978 1 921966 41 5

Design and typesetting by Big Cat Design
Diagrams on pp. 42, 43 and 58 courtesy of Shutterstock
Typeset in Sabon 11/17pt
Printed in Shenzhen, China, by Ink Asia

This book uses paper sourced under ISO 14001 guidelines from
well-managed forests and other controlled sources.

10 9 8 7 6 5 4 3 2 1

Disclaimer
While this book is intended as a general information resource
and all care has been taken in compiling the contents, this book
does not take account of individual circumstances and is not in
any way a substitute for professional advice. Neither the author
nor the publisher and their distributors can be held responsible
for any loss, claim or action that may arise from reliance on the
information contained in this book.

To Zach and Samuel, my reason for living and my vulnerability to life.

Thank you to Don and my whole family — we have had our bumps in the road but every one has led us to the wonderment we enjoy! And thank you to my friends for the positivity we bounce between us.

Contents

Introduction *1*

1 **Healthy eating** *5*

2 **It all started with a theory** *14*

3 **Who or what is at the helm?** *38*

4 **Learning and its effect on food choice** *86*

5 **Changing behaviours** *101*

6 **Eating, emotions, personality and motivation** *134*

7 **Media and marketing** *155*

8 **Food labelling** *168*

9 **Making changes** *179*

Appendix 1: Dutch Eating Behaviour Questionnaire *183*

Appendix 2: Intuitive Eating Scale *189*

Resources *193*

Endnotes *197*

Bibliography *204*

Index *212*

Introduction

You may have read a little or even a lot about healthy eating. Either way, you're likely to find *Change the Way You Eat* goes well beyond the traditional nutrition and diet topics. In this book you won't find definitions and examples of nutrients and energy. Instead you're going to be exposed to a bit of theory and research on why we eat what we eat, and you'll discover that much of this lies in the realm of psychology. Calculating calories, grams of this or that is not directly relevant, and in fact as we will see it's not overly helpful anyway, which explains why it seems many efforts to improve community eating have been largely unsuccessful.

Change the Way You Eat won't tell you how to get slim and stay slim, but hopefully it will motivate you to set your own path and stay on track to your health goals. You're about to launch into an exploration of the processes (both hidden and obvious) that exert influence over our desire to eat and our control of how much we eat. Uncovering these processes may just be part of our health salvation, by ourselves, for ourselves. This book is more about the psychology of eating than nutrition. It's a revealing tale: our love affair with fat and salt, our battle against innate desires, the seduction of marketing, and the triumph of common sense over habit. Such is food psychology.

Introduction to food psychology

A few years ago you wouldn't have seen a lot of information around in the area of food psychology; indeed, you would have been forgiven for thinking there wasn't much happening in the way of research in this area, but that's not the case. For decades researchers have been studying what makes us eat more or less. For example, researchers in the 1980s quickly realised that not only did we eat more at a buffet, but even putting high-calorie food out of reach didn't deter us from adding it to our brimming plates.[1] Just why this information hasn't made it to us one can only guess. Maybe it's a fear of the masses realising that food production might not, by and large, have our best interests at heart. It's rarely good when the 'troops revolt'.

Nonetheless there are gaps in our understanding, and the more answers we seek the more questions arise. And, of course, while much of this knowledge has been circulating in university halls it clearly hasn't made it into the mainstream (though marketing and advertising have been onto it for a while). So boning up on this fascinating area will not only change the way you think about food, weight and food production, it will also provide you with hours of dinner conversation, as you will find you have knowledge that few hold under their belts, even many 'experts'.

Before we launch ourselves headlong into eating inhibitions and satiety, let's just take a moment to acknowledge that studying behaviour is not easily done. If you undertake research in a laboratory then this can confound results; likewise if you study in a natural setting, numerous confounding variables can occur which can't be controlled. The science of studying behaviour is very complex with hundreds of factors affecting any behaviour, which also makes it more difficult to reproduce studies so that a clear and more consistent pattern can be discerned. Psychology is also heavily weighted in theory, so yes you will get a number of theories thrown at you and if history tells us anything it's that most of these theories hold up for most people but not all, and eventually some smarter theories will add to or amend the original. So, like life, our ideas about food and eating continually change, and that's a good thing!

Why understand food psychology?

Understanding why we eat what we eat is essential to anyone who wants to lead a healthier life, as well as those who work in the area of health and nutrition. But more importantly it's essential that we recognise our early internal mechanisms, for ourselves and for our children, for they are an important key to our self-determination and control.

I have a personal belief, based on strong anecdotal evidence, that too many of us focus on numbers as the answer to disordered eating and being overweight — focusing on calories of this and that, grams of this and that, points here and there and so on. Yet in many cases this can simply detract from the real issue, as it almost obscures our responsibility and role in our own eating habits. Healthy eating is a lifestyle we adopt and something we should all fully understand. Healthy eating is about having an almost sixth sense of what constitutes a healthy meal or food, so much so that you can pick the imposters a mile away. You don't need to be distracted by numbers. To my mind, numbers are a scapegoat or a red herring. A colleague mentioned to me one day that a friend of hers was on a popular diet but still ate McDonald's twice a week because doing so didn't tip her over her allowed points. Now there is nothing wrong in having the odd takeaway if you have a predominantly healthy diet, but this sort of trade-off tends to suggest that the healthy food is second best and something to be bartered. We need to rethink our attitude towards healthy eating. Take, for example, a bill you have to pay. Look at just one of the numbers on the sheet. What does that tell you about the underlying actions that led to this bill? That's right: nothing. In isolation it tells you nothing. It's like building a house: you have to have a great frame in place before you finetune the home. Understanding healthy eating principles of quality, timing, variety, portions, body cues and dynamism (flexibility) is, I believe, far more effective in permanent change than counting calories and grams.

Needless to say, if you are a health professional, understanding food psychology will enable you to better create eating plans with clients and work effectively and realistically with supporting your clients in achieving their eating habit goals. However, nutrition psychology in its journey to the 'outer world' may well mean that you will be challenged on the traditional paradigm of the expert–client approach. After all, there isn't a great deal of evidence to suggest this has been a particularly successful approach; the new wave of research supports the client-centred approach as being the most effective.

As you begin to read this book it's a great idea to have a highlighting pen handy. Most sections will provide you with information you will relate to. Highlight the eating habits and choices that relate to you, those that you feel need improvement. At regular points throughout the book there are tasks and strategies you can reflect on and decide if you want to apply them to yourself. Having already highlighted the areas of concern you can simply go back to these sections and use them as your focus for change.

Consume, savour, reflect, absorb and build!

LEANNE COOPER

1
Healthy Eating

It's likely you don't need to be convinced of the virtues of healthy eating, but if you needed any further proof here's something to mull over. Studies show that poor nutrition can impair not only our daily health and wellbeing but also our longevity and long-term quality of life. Poor nutrition can affect our:

- ability to cope with life and stressors
- level of energy and ability to be active
- risk of ill-health and disease including excess weight, high blood pressure, heart disease, high (bad) cholesterol, diabetes, bone disease, some cancers, tooth decay, mental illness and more.

Conversely, eating well can provide you with:

- feelings of wellbeing and vitality
- increased lifespan and quality of life

- **improved health and reduced risk of illness**
- **increased capacity to cope with life.**

In other words, eating well can improve your mind, body and we may well argue it's just darn good for the soul!

It's also important to consider how we relate to food, and to remind ourselves that food is about nourishment and enjoyment. So many of us see food in a defeating way; for example, some view food as:

- **a reward or punishment**
- **a set of numbers and targets**
- **being related to our self-esteem**
- **something we need in order to cope with life's challenges.**

Food and eating is about health and happiness. The two are not separate — to a degree our happiness depends on our eating habits and choices. We should be able to freely choose foods we wish to eat yet have an almost unconscious appreciation for how much we need and what foods we need (and what foods we simply want).

Consider the current emphasis on the issue of our growing waistlines and the resulting health challenges. The current tendency is to view the answer as a diet, that we need to count calories, restrain ourselves, punish ourselves, categorise ourselves and so on. But few recognise the loss of connection with the food we choose and decide to eat; few also are aware of our body's cues for hunger and satiety, that we need to know what these are and recognise and respond appropriately to them.

What is a good diet?

An elusive question: what constitutes a 'good' diet? Let's look at some of the principles that go towards the creation of a healthful diet. We'll also take some lessons from the diets of populations who live to a ripe old age.

Three basic principles can ensure that a diet is nutritionally sound. These are variety, wholesomeness and unprocessed food. Two other factors should also be taken into account: a consideration of individual circumstances that may vary nutritional requirements; and a 'dynamic' or flexible approach to eating. We'll look at each of these factors in turn.

Variety is truly the spice of life!

The importance of making sure a diet is continually varied to include a wide variety of food cannot be overstated. Food should be selected from a wide variety of sources each day, as diets that exclude several food groups are associated with an increased risk of chronic disease and mortality. Eating a wide variety of nutritious foods is important in four ways:

1. Eating from a variety of food groups every day is highly likely to result in a diet that provides ample amounts of each of the nutrients essential for good health. It is not necessary to eat from each food group at every meal.

2. Because foods within the same food group contain different nutrients, it is important to consume a variety of foods within each group. Fruit is a good example: strawberries are rich in vitamin C, whereas bananas are rich in a number of B-group vitamins. Similarly, red meat provides more dietary iron than other members of the same food group. Therefore, eating a wide variety of food ensures you are obtaining the largest possible range of

nutrients from your diet. By selecting a variety of foods each day, over the week and at different times of the year, you have a much greater chance of obtaining enough of all of the nutrients your body requires for health and wellbeing.

3. Eating a variety of foods from different biological origins can benefit health. For example:

   ■ Some saturated fatty acids appear to raise blood cholesterol levels that contribute to the development of coronary heart disease, but polyunsaturated fats can actively reduce blood cholesterol levels. Choosing foods from different biological sources (both animal and vegetable) ensures a variety of fats in the diet and a balance of the different types of fat.

   ■ Dietary fibre from oats has been associated with a reduction in blood cholesterol while dietary fibre from wheat prevents constipation.

   ■ Cruciferous vegetables (including broccoli, cabbage, cauliflower, brussels sprouts and bok choy) are thought to contain specific substances said to assist in the prevention of a number of cancers.

4. No food is guaranteed to be entirely free of substances that, in excess, may be harmful to the body. For example, strawberries might contain a specific contaminant and bananas another, therefore alternating fruit choices will reduce the risk of ingesting too much of one particular contaminant.

Tip: **Research is fairly clear that a healthy diet will provide better health outcomes than almost any supplement.**

As we'll see soon, research into antioxidants, dietary habits and supplements consistently comes back to food being a safe and more potent factor in longevity and good health.

Wholesomeness — not reduced parts

The term 'wholesome' food generally refers to the variety of food that is made from whole ingredients. For example, wholegrain bread contains the goodness of the entire grain, rather than the highly processed flour that is used to make some white bread. A good diet should rely primarily on food that is wholesome and remains as similar as possible to its original state; this ensures that the diet is rich in important nutrients and will also limit any possible contamination from food preservatives, colours and flavours.

Unprocessed food

An ideal diet should not rely heavily on processed food such as tinned, pre-prepared food, fast food, reheated food and so on. As a general rule, the less processed a food is, the greater its nutrient content. Additionally, the less a food is processed, the fewer preservatives, colours, flavours and additives it contains.

Individuality

In addition to these principles it is important to remember that an individual's nutritional needs are dependent on a range of interacting factors including genetic, environmental, social, psychological, and other lifestyle factors such as physical activity. Therefore, a healthy diet alone is certainly not enough to guarantee optimal health. Additionally, simply eating all the food groups in the right balance does not ensure your diet is ideal. A range of factors can all impact significantly on an individual's nutritional requirements. These include:

- **digestion and absorption**
- **sensitivities and allergies**
- **medications currently being used**
- **quality, cost and availability of food**
- **age, health and lifestyle.**

Dynamic

A way of eating, or if you wish 'diet', is dynamic and can adjust to changes in an individual's life; such changes allow for the vast differences between us. It is very unlikely that any one 'diet' will suit all people. Most diets will sit well with some people for a while and we can often get something from diets in terms of being exposed to other foods and ways of eating, but in the end most commonly they fail and leave us feeling disappointed, sometimes with ourselves.

How can we know what the best way of eating is?

The question no doubt burning in your mind is 'Which foods pack the greatest health punch?' This is where we start to see a pattern emerge. If, for example, we take the diets of communities who live the longest, such as those in Okinawa, Japan, we note the heavy representation of vegetables in their diet, providing a variety of phytonutrients, antioxidants and flavonoids (you can see these in

Table 1 on p. 12). Their diet is low in red meat but high in fish and also rich in 'functional foods' such as herbs and spices.[1]

Sardinia (Italy) in the Mediterranean also comes up trumps in regards to the average life expectancy and here again we see a high intake of vegetables and fruit, legumes and complex carbohydrates, some fish and healthy oils and fats. In fact it has been confirmed that such diets significantly reduce mortality rates (from all causes including stroke and cognitive impairment).[2]

Seeing the pattern? Yes, plant foods are a recurring factor in healthful diets! Not only do they tend to represent the most nutrient-diverse and nutrient-dense foods, but further support for their positive effect is evident in the diets of those who live longest. The consumption of fish, too, appears to be an important factor in health and longevity.

Where are we in the scheme of things?

If you feel that the current stock of messages and strategies has been ineffective in reducing our waistlines or improving our eating habits, you are probably right. Despite decades of effort going into addressing overweight and obesity, many developed countries are getting fatter. Having said that, there does appear to be a trend of some Western countries towards a plateau in overweight numbers, however, it is early days so just what this is attributable to is not yet clear. On the downside, our many nutritionally devoid manufactured foods are now making their way onto the stage in developing countries, so much so that we see countries such as Mexico now second only to the United States in obesity rates and some South American nations' rates of obesity increasing faster than most places in the world.

Table 1: Obesity rates in the OECD for adults (percentage of population)[3]

	Males	Females	Total % of pop.
United Kingdom	23.9	22.1	23.0
Canada	23.2	25.2	24.2
Australia	23.6	25.5	24.6
Chile	30.7	19.2	25.1
New Zealand	27.0	26.0	25.5
Mexico	34.5	24.0	30.0
United States	35.5	32.2	33.8

How is your country faring?

Australia has seen a rise in overweight and obesity in adults since 1995 (that was the last national nutrition survey), from 56.3 per cent of those aged eighteen and over being overweight or obese to 61.2 per cent in 2007–8 and 62.8 per cent in 2011–12. On a more positive note, the rates in children aged five to seventeen increased from 20.9 per cent to 24.7 per cent in 2007–8 but remained stable to 2012.

If you have any doubt at all that obesity and childhood obesity is a challenge to our community consider the following:

- In Australia, 60 per cent of adults and 25 per cent of kids are overweight or obese. To put this in perspective, consider a family dinner with ten members around the table; six of those adults and one in four of the children will be overweight or obese.

- Countries such as England, Switzerland, Korea and Italy have seen a plateau in their rates of obesity, with Spain and France having shown modest increases in obesity.

The United States, Ireland and Canada have shown much greater increases.[4]

■ The total health cost for obesity in the United States in 2008 was estimated at US$147 billion — that's *billion*.[5]

■ According to OECD research at least one in two of us (from half of the OECD countries) is overweight or obese.[6]

■ Being obese as a child increases the likelihood of being obese as an adult, and childhood obesity has been shown to increase the risk of early death in adulthood. Keep in mind, though, that not all obese adults were overweight or obese as children. Having said that, once a child becomes overweight or obese it is less likely that they will remedy this without intervention.

■ The World Health Organization (2010) suggests that some 5 per cent of global mortality can be attributed to obesity.

■ In 2003 having a high body mass was thought to have been the cause of 7.5 per cent of disease and injury in Australia. This sits behind only tobacco (7.8 per cent) and high blood pressure (7.6 per cent).

Statistics are a great tool to really ensure a message hits home, and I am sure you get the picture. But while many countries are still struggling, others are making some headway. Clearly there is a way forward and there are some trailblazers to take note of.

Change the Way You Eat is your key to becoming your own trailblazer. It's your opportunity to create a healthful lifestyle that suits your needs, one that goes beyond trends or perhaps is the very start of one. Well done to you for taking the first step of many on this exciting road!

2
It all started with a theory

B efore we launch into just what makes us eat too much or why we almost go weak at the knees when the dessert menu arrives, let's draw attention to the multitude of influences affecting our final decision 'to eat or not to eat'. Food choices involve factors ranging from our life stage (for example teenagers' eating choices will differ from those of their parents) through to our personal beliefs such as vegetarianism, and social influences, not the least of which is advertising.

The Furst Model of Food Choice was indeed one of the 'first' theoretical food models on the scene, and is our 'picture that paints a thousand words'. Schematically it represents the factors behind our food choices so that we can grasp the detail without losing sight of the broader picture. To demonstrate the model we will use a family of four (who differ in age, gender, beliefs, financial resources and so on).

Why are models important?
Theoretical models provide us with the opportunity to understand in a very visual way factors that influence us and the way in which we

behave around food. In the case of food choice models they become an exposé on a wide range of factors that have power over how we make food choices. Food models highlight influences that:

- **might seem logical, but are worth seeing in black and white, such as the effect our family situation has over our eating habits**

- **are a little more subtle and often need a direct beam of light so that we can be more mindful, for example marketing and advertising**

- **most of us really have no real conscious awareness of, for example social settings, including the number of people, placement of food and even the music playing when we are shopping or dining out.**

Theories, particularly those that can be shown diagrammatically, are also excellent ways of showing you how interconnected and complex the picture of something so seemingly simple can be (though, as we will see, not losing sight of the big picture is just as important), and also how very individual it is. For these reasons, looking at a food model is important, as it forms a solid platform of knowledge from which to appreciate and explore the more practical information later in the book.

For those of you working in the health or wellbeing field you will also be wise to become familiar with at least the more well-known models as they are commonly used in planning and in creating health strategies, surveys and in research design. If you ever plan on working within a government agency or in community health, being familiar with the most common health models is essential so you can 'talk the talk'.

But Furst ... the model of food choice

You have probably never given it much thought, but every decision you make in choosing any particular food or beverage involves numerous factors, ranging from access, price, quality, appearance, brand and so on. But you can be sure that there are a whole lot of people who have spent a great deal of time on this and many are cashing in on your thought processes, regardless of how unconscious they may be on your part.

You may not have felt your food choices are of any great relevance but they are of interest to a wide range of professionals including health departments, nutritionists, food outlets, food stores and marketing and advertising agencies.

There is a great deal of merit in being a mindful shopper, consumer and eater. Potentially, mindful eating puts you as the consumer back in control. Mindless eating, on the other hand, may result in you being a victim to marketing insofar as mindless consumption is far more easily impressed and led. Conscious eating, as we will see, is likely to be a very great 'weapon' in our arsenal against unhealthy eating practices and excess weight. We'll look at this in a lot more detail soon.

Take a look at Figure 1, the Furst Model of Food Choice (p. 18). Don't be put off by all the arrows and labels — it's actually much simpler than you might think. Let's break it down. The model has many layers representing the many factors governing our food choices.

1. At the top is our life course (or stage of life), for example infancy, school child, adolescence, student, professional, first-time parent, empty nester, retired, to mention just a few.

2. Depending on our stage of life we can be influenced by numerous factors including our ideals, personal factors

such as age or gender, resources we have access to such as money and education, social factors (religion, for example) and contextual factors such as the atmosphere when eating at a restaurant.

3. Moving down the layers, we come to 'personal system'. Quite simply, this is how each of these layers above come together and lead us to getting closer to our ultimate decision, to eat or not to eat!

4. Inching ever closer to the final choice, we come to value negotiations. This is where those two voices (the angel and the devil) in our head are whispering (sometimes one is yelling), urging us to reward ourselves for running such a tight ship and pop that mouth-watering packet of chocolate biscuits in the trolley even if the budget is still tight.

5. This leads us to strategies, the formulation of ideas used to come to a decision.

6. And at last, the choice!

It's rather convenient not to think of food so consciously at times and, yes, of course these decision-making processes are so much faster than how you have just read above. They occur almost instantly. But is that such a good thing? Perhaps slowing down for a moment and considering the basis for wanting a food might be good for us. We don't need to labour over every single morsel that passes our lips, but rather, we can stop at some point in the day (or week or month) and bring into awareness our eating habits.

When I was studying psychology a lecturer told us that sometimes events or issues in our lives aren't to be fixed, but rather just acknowledged for what they were, and that today they are not and needn't be as they were. In other words, re-evaluating the way we do things, not seeing things as broken and instead choosing not to do what simply doesn't work for us, can be a great remedy and internal power. It's a bit like reprogramming and, as we will see, many of our eating habits are ingrained and a number of these may need a tweak.

Figure 1: The Furst Model of Food Choice[1]

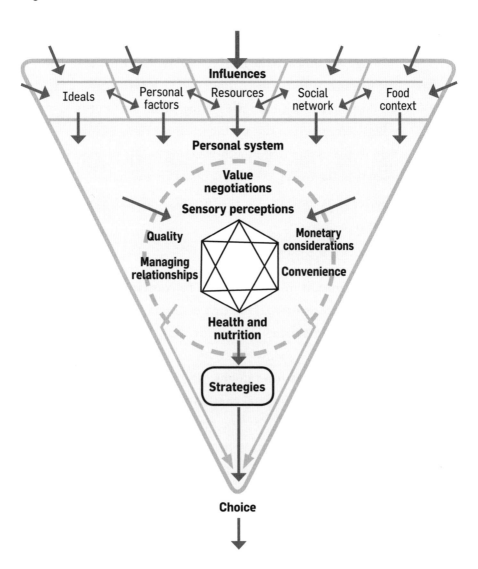

Your life stage influences

What life stage are you at? Just have a think for a moment. Consider other members in your household or even those around you — what life stage are they at? Most likely the factors that affect your food choices will differ from those around you. For example, in your home there may be a newly returned-to-work mother, a tradesperson father, a high school child and a university student, with a retired grandparent. Clearly, these people will be influenced by different factors — some will be affected by peers and others not, some by resources such as money and others not so directly.

It can seem as if our behaviour changes over time. However, as we develop, our behaviour simply tends to become more consolidated and broader while the core remains reasonably consistent. Research suggests, though, that there are certain life stages that seem to pave the way for change, including alterations in food choices. In some cases this can be very handy, namely:

- **during adolescence, being a transition from childhood to adulthood, hence why some fussy foodies suddenly drop the near-gagging act at the sight of a vegetable and will eat almost anything**

- **during stressful periods and major life events such as moving, divorce, major illness, changing school or profession, known periods where fundamental behaviours can alter.**

- **Most of us will also know of someone who has totally changed their life after a brush with cancer or a death in the family.**

Influences

There are a range of factors exerting power over our food choices. Such factors can be within our control, such as our ideals, while others may be beyond our control, such as cost. In fact, some types of influence may fall into more than one category, for example socioeconomic status (that is, how much we earn, our jobs, where we live and so on) may fall into personal factors as well as resources.

Let's take a more detailed look at some of these influences.

IDEALS

We all have ideals, principles and values we hold that move us to pursue our goals or to direct us in life along a path. We largely learn our ideals while we are growing up, while we are being 'socialised'. A really good example is the ideal of 'table manners' — though just what counts as table manners differs between cultures, life stages and so on.

PERSONAL FACTORS

Clearly we have our own specific set of personal characteristics that make us who we are and set us apart from each other. In food choice there can be many ways in which we differ from others. Some of our differences include:

- **physiology, for example our perception of taste and smell, even our genetics will 'flavour' our food choices**

- **emotional states such as our mood, fears and phobias**

- **psychological factors such as our self-concept or who we believe we are.**

Healthful eating task:
What food-related ideals do you hold?

Task 1: Now you have a picture of distinctions between different life stages, try to define your 'food ideals'. From the list below, circle or write down some of the ideals that are important to you. To you, food should be:

Safe and clean

Healthy

Meet my nutrient needs

A home brand (a store's own brand)

From a brand I trust

Liked by my children

Convenient and easy to access

Healthy for children

Inexpensive

Tasty

Nutritious

Priced well

Better if a famous person eats it

Anything but a home brand

A brand I like

Available at my local store

Considerate of the environment

Long lasting

From sources that do not harm animals

Vegetarian

Popular foods

A good source of energy

Unique foods

Only current season foods

Easy to cook

Easy to prepare

Easy to make into a meal

Low in sugar

Low in salt

High in fibre

Low in fat

High in protein

Now consider how the factors you have selected affect your eating habits and routines. How many are choices made because of the way you were brought up? And how many have you adopted by choice? How are your ideals influenced by advertising?

Task 2: Is there an ideal you have noted which you would like to give up or change so that you can have healthier eating habits? If 'yes', write this down on a piece of paper, and describe what ideal will replace it if there needs to be one. Try to use as few words as possible so it's more of a picture. Now place this on your fridge (so you see it regularly). Each day, look at this note at least once and ask yourself where it has cropped up. Tell yourself, 'Tomorrow I won't do that'. Do this for seven days or until you begin to notice you no longer hold that eating ideal, but ensure you practise this for at least a month (once each a day) so that you can be more assured that you have reprogrammed your brain.

It's thought that we develop our personal eating habits in relation to our self-concept or identity and that our eating habits reflect who we are. Once again we can see that there is likely to be a strong social learning aspect involved.

Let's now explore an example where we can see these factors playing out in real life. Ever heard that if you are overweight the only way to lose weight is to go on a diet? Yes! Let's take a look at a common ideal that all too often grows from personal factors: the belief that dieting is the route to weight control. If we think about this assertion for a moment we can see that underlying it are ideals and personal factors (many of which we will soon see are self-defeating and work against us), not the least being that:

- **being thin is healthy**
- **dieting is the only way to control my weight**
- **eating less will help me to lose weight**
- **if I am overweight I must eat less**
- **if I am overweight I need a diet.**

Sound familiar? Recognise the ideals and the personal characteristics in the above statements?

So what does the research say? An interesting study in the United States looked at the differences between lean, overweight and obese women in the way they selected food. It seems that, at least in this study, overweight and obese women were more influenced by the cost of food; in addition they saw themselves as more emotional and more likely to eat as a consequence of their emotions and have a much greater liking for food generally, and for fatty options. Interestingly, both groups were equally influenced by taste when choosing foods.[2]

Another great example is dieting amongst teens. We know that dieting and food restriction (referred to in clinical literature as weight control behaviours) is common amongst teens. All too often this happens as a consequence of personal factors of weight concerns, body image and body dissatisfaction. Interestingly, studies show these behaviours are strongly predictive of increases in body fat in later life.[3] But wait, there's more. The same studies show that skipping meals may not be the answer either. Young girls who eat breakfast and dinner are less likely to be overweight when they are older. Clearly some of our values and personal characteristics can get in the way of a healthy life.

This is not to say that some of our ideals and personal characteristics are not a positive influence. A personal trainer who holds fitness and healthy eating as important personal characteristics will be driven to pursue both, as might a mother who values offering her children foods free from additives.

RESOURCES

How often do you put in an online order to have your organic meat and produce sent directly to your home? Some of you might be saying 'every week', but it's likely most will be saying 'what?'. Not all of us have the resources to shop in this way: it takes time, money, access to such services and so on. And there you have it — 'resources' explained in a nutshell. In short, resources can be defined as the tools and assets at our disposal that we use to access food. This includes money, location, equipment, space, mobility, skills, education, training, information and support. The degree to which these affect our food choices will depend on a number of factors including our socio-economic status.

A great study conducted in Victoria, Australia, called the Victorian Lifestyle and Neighbourhood Study, or VicLANES for short, demonstrates clearly that there is a strong link between where we live and what we eat. VicLANES found that those living in a high socio-economic area in Victoria were more likely to:

- buy groceries that were low in fat, salt and sugar, and high in fibre
- purchase fruit
- exercise at levels sufficient for health
- spend time walking.[4]

And it's probably no surprise to you that they also found that fast food outlets are more common in low to mid socio-economic areas, hence those living in these areas were also more likely to buy and consume fast foods. In addition, VicLANES highlighted that men from lower socio-economic areas were more likely to consume alcohol at a level that could cause short-term health issues.

Resources are great if you are one of the 'haves' — not so much if you aren't. This might be logical, and certainly easy to identify, but it's much harder to close the social divide.

SOCIAL FRAMEWORK

Who do you hang out with? Where do you spend your free time? Your answer might range from family and friends through to church or cultural groups, activist groups, sporting teams, political or social agencies, workmates and so on. Your answers make up your social framework; it is likely there will be a number of groups and settings, and each may colour how you chose what you eat. Your social framework is the part of your life where you mix with others and this influences the person you are.

Perhaps this is a generalisation but it would be no surprise to find that a person who is environmentally and health conscious and loves animals is also vegetarian. Their social framework of being involved in 'green' activities, animal rights and health, is consistent with the likelihood they don't eat animal flesh.

FOOD CONTEXT

If you run a restaurant or other food outlet you will find some very interesting snippets about how to get people to linger longer, spend more or buy want you want to sell (mind you, your customers reading this book won't be so susceptible!). The food environment (of which there are many ranging from home, canteens, restaurants, supermarkets and so on) exerts an enormous effect over your food choices and consumption. Ever noticed that there is now music pumping through many stores, including the supermarket? It's not just there to make the weekly shop feel less tiresome. It's designed to make you shop longer, feel carefree and hopefully buy more.

A range of contextual factors affect our food choices and intake, including:

- **the type and range of food choices on offer**

- **meal context, for example the type of meal and its contents, temperature, appearance**

- **social context, for example the social occasion, how appealing the environment is**

- **the environment, for example where we eat and the surroundings**

- **the presence of others, which affects how much we eat.**

Don't you just love the extra effort a restaurant goes to when they have a candle lit at your dinner table? Not only does that dim lighting seem to help you relax but miraculously you can fit in a dessert you wouldn't normally be inclined to eat or an extra drink or two. One of the prolific researchers in food psychology is Brian Wansink. Along with Pierre Chandon, Wansink reviewed the literature on factors that affect food choices. Here are just a few findings they found to be consistent.

- **Dim, soft lighting seems to get us eating for longer and consequently just that little bit more. Apparently soft lighting makes us feel more comfortable and is a disinhibitor (put plainly, it stops us from having self-control).**

- **Nice aromas from food and cooking, even if we aren't conscious of them, appear to make us want to eat and drink more also.**

- **Soft music makes us eat more slowly, have longer meals and eat and drink more. Just like the lighting, appealing music can have the effect of acting as a disinhibitor, encouraging us to eat and drink a little extra.**

- **Apparently music can create positive feelings that encourage us to linger, but can also alter our perception of just how long we have been eating (or shopping, for that matter).**

- **Music that is familiar and liked, and has a slower tempo, encourages us to shop just a little longer, hence those catchy hits played in the supermarket.**

- **Even the actual utensils we use to dish up our food affect our eating, with larger containers and plates tending to encourage us to consume more.**

- **Interestingly, an empty plate signals to many of us to stop eating, so having someone continually add to your plate or glass simply encourages us to eat and/or drink more than we actually need to.[5]**

The authors suggest that distraction may be playing an important role in these results. Supporting this are studies that show watching TV while eating dinner not only causes us to eat more but also interferes with our ability to reflect on just how much we have eaten. Although, interestingly, the nature of a TV commercial, for example, be it funny, sad, boring and so on, doesn't seem to affect the volume of food we eat.[6]

It seems that eating while we are distracted (sometimes referred to as mindless eating) also interferes with our signals of being full. In fact, distraction works on a deep level according to Chandon and Wansink. It leads to greater intake of food by influencing our taste perception and feelings; that is, it leads us to feeling more positive about the food and leaves our actual physiological states (such as cues of fullness) out in the cold. We will look at the area of body signals as a clue to establishing healthy eating habits soon, as we'll see it's a central factor in permanent change. In fact, there is a strong shift away from diet-centred approaches to health towards healthy eating-centred approaches, which empower people to be reflective about their eating and choices, to enjoy food and not fear it and to listen to their body cues again. More on this soon!

Indeed, if you look over the research in this area there are a huge amount of studies. Some of the interesting findings from this research include:

- Just watching others eat makes us want to eat more.

- We eat more when we are served more food, regardless of our body size or the food served — portion size has a strong effect.[7] Perhaps it's that 'waste not, want not' adage?

- The easier it is for us to access food, the more likely we are to consume it and consume more of it.

- The longer a meal takes, the more we will tend to consume. So watch out for those five-course meals ...

- The more people we eat with, the more we tend to eat.

Healthful eating task:
Food context

Take a moment to review the food context section and circle or highlight the factors that you particularly relate to and feel you need to improve on. Start with just one or two actions at first — they may be easy ones or ones that you are really passionate about. Either way, write them out on a piece of paper, then write out your strategy for change for each. Start out small and ensure your strategies are achievable. Now place this 'action sheet' on the fridge or any other prominent place. Each time you see your action sheet, reflect on your previous attempts to see how you are going and if you need to tweak anything; self-appraisal is a very important part of change.

Strategies to reduce mindless eating and increase healthy eating habits can include the following:

- **Use smaller plates for your meals.**
- **Serve foods with smaller utensils; even a dessert spoon is better than a ladle-type spoon.**
- **Shop only from a list or order online.**
- **Place treats at the back of the fridge or cupboard.**
- **Ensure healthy snacks are always on hand and place them at the front of the fridge or cupboard.**
- **Avoid buffet-style restaurants — if you like this type of restaurant, limit your visits to once a month.**

- When you do go to a buffet, select just two dishes first and avoid mounds of food. Low and flat servings are best.

- Sit at a table away from the buffet so you aren't continually exposed to huge amounts of varied dishes.

- Don't let the wait staff clear your table, so you can see how many servings you have consumed.

- Likewise, leave remnants of food (such as bones) on your plate to remind you of how much you have consumed.

- Start eating last — enjoy conversation and your surroundings first, then enjoy your food more thoughtfully.

- Leave just a small portion of food on your plate to avoid your host offering you more.

- Consider how much you will eat before you begin, rather than eating as you go. It can help to be mindful of how hungry you are before you start out.

Practise these each day or as often as they occur. You will need to do this for the pivotal time of one month and potentially keep practising for some time. Often it's two steps forward, one step back, but always focus on the positives you have created.

We will come back to this list in more detail soon, but for now it gives you something to put into practice at this early stage so you get a real feel for this non-diet approach.

Personal system

Now that we are a little familiar with some common terms and concepts encountered when looking at eating habits, let's take a look at the next level in our model to help bring it all together. Personal systems are thought processes (cognitive processes) that bring our choices into action; in other words, they are our thinking put into practice.

As you wander along the supermarket aisle and stop miraculously at the chocolate section one part of you thinks, 'Oh, yes, chocolate'. Your immediate answer might be, 'No I don't need it' to which the hungry beast inside you says, 'But you've been really good, you haven't had any for weeks and you've been to the gym — go on.' And before you know it that chocolate bar sits a little guiltily in your trolley (dark chocolate, though, with all those lovely antioxidant flavonoids, might counteract some of the guilt). What you have just done in that instance is known as a value negotiation, using your personal systems to come to a decision about whether to purchase chocolate and which type.

While such food decisions might sound like a lengthy process, it's the value negotiations and strategies we use (which we will look at next) that make these decisions generally unconscious and very fast. Our value negotiations are often hierarchical: we have certain values that we prize over others. For example, if I have diabetes it's likely I will value low-GI foods, perhaps even over taste or cost. Having said that, it is good to remember that often not all our values can be satisfied, which is why they tend to be hierarchical.

Understanding your value negotiations can be a very revealing exercise and also useful in amending habits that could serve you better if they were more positive. Complete the following task to help you assess your strategies for choosing foods.

Healthful eating task:
Uncover your value negotiations

Consider two foods that you enjoy: one a healthy option, for example something fresh and unprocessed; the other a less healthy option, such as a type of junk food. Now answer the following questions, making sure to write down your answers.

1. **What priorities encourage you to opt for the healthier option? What priorities encourage you to choose the less healthy option? Think about what it is that each option gives you and what makes you purchase each option.**

2. **At what times do you eat the unhealthy option? What contextual and personal factors are involved? What is your mood or emotion at the time?**

3. **Consider your responeses above. How can you use them to create a strategy to reduce the consumption of an unhealthy food? And, how can you use the value negotiations to support your healthy food choices more broadly? Don't beat yourself up, you are using a positive action to do something more positive — it's not about guilt!**

Food choice strategies

The way in which we prioritise our food values and the factors we use to make a final decision helps to make the process much simpler. In other words, strategies such as plans, rules, routines and so on simplify our food selection process. Now food choice strategies are an interesting area, and if you are in the business of selling food or marketing and advertising, this area will be of special interest. Understanding food choice strategies opens the door to selling more of your product. For example, early research indicated that we tend to shop at eye level — that is, we are far more likely to buy products at our eye level on the shelves. 'Shelf location' is therefore much sought after and consequently stores can charge a premium for manufacturers to place their products at eye level (unless your product appeals to children, then it is likely to cost more to place it at the counter).

Consumer researchers have spent a great deal of time and money understanding our shopping 'scripts': what you do, what you think when comparing a brand, if you shop from habit, what those habits are and why, what priorities you use to decide between brands, what you feel as you enter the shop, how long you stay, where you look, where you go to first and why you're in a shop. This might seem quite boring to most of us, but bringing out these unconscious acts is a marketer's therapy session.

Keep in mind that as our lives change so do our food choice strategies, so unlike our values they are more malleable, which is good news to advertisers. They also change from one situation to another; for example, we use a different script for food shopping to clothes shopping.

Shopping habits are also commonly of use to food coaches, nutritionists and others who work with eating habits. The benefits of understanding the underlying factors that influence our food choices and how they meld together to bring us to a final decision include:

- identifying values and beliefs that lead to unhealthy food choices
- identifying habits that lead to less desirable food choices
- highlighting where changes and tweaking are required and where to focus attention in terms of creating new programs for healthy eating habits
- allowing health professionals to recognise the more intimate factors that lead people to food choices while still seeing the larger picture of dietary sufficiency
- bringing conscious focus for clients on the behaviours that don't serve them well; it's important that we are all active participants in both the uncovering of our challenges as well as in creating the process of moving forward.

You can also apply 'scripts' to eating out (we'll come back to this in Chapter 7 when we look at the effect of marketing on food choice and eating habits).

Healthful eating task:
Know your shopping habits

Given your home should be by and large full of healthful foods, let's focus attention on this area by writing out a food shopping script. However, for those who eat out more than they cook it might be beneficial to review an eating-out script.

Write out your food shopping script. Include everything — where you park (or if you walk or cycle); which aisles you go down and which you avoid or never venture down, and why; if you use a list; what happens if you go shopping at different times; if you shop differently when hungry; if you buy by brand items or home brand (a store's own brand); if you rush or take your time; which aisles you spend most and least time in, and why; how you pack your shopping; where you place it when you get home, and why.

Now review your script. Try to pick out good habits and behaviours and ones you would like to adapt. You may need to consider:

- **if you shop out of habit**

- **if you spend more time in aisles containing less healthy options**

- **if you read labels**

- **if you use the shopping list or if you also buy random foods that are needed.**

Also think about which foods you value over others (you can determine these by the time taken to consider them, how they are packed, where they are in your home and so on). Review who you are shopping for apart from yourself, and what it is the food is providing for them. Is it pacifying children or feeding them? Are your choices focused on one or two individuals while you overlook yourself? And so on.

Is there a pattern of healthy choices you need to foster and is there a less healthful pattern you need to be conscious of? You may need to alter your shopping habits, which aisles you go down, and what your priorities are for food.

Finally, list three things you believe are healthful habits and then three things that are less healthful that you would like to change. Alongside each, list one way you could alter this behaviour next time you go to buy food. Place your list with each shopping list for the next month or until you have made these changes permanent. Keep in mind your habits will resist attempts to change so keep self-evaluating how you are going.

3
Who or what is at the helm?

Ultimately, just who is calling the shots when it comes to our food choices and intake? Is it the food itself? After all, there certainly seem to be some foods attractively packaged that beg us to eat them. Is it our own internal factors, our tastebuds, energy requirements or even genetics? Or is it our personality? Who doesn't know someone who turns over every packet in the cupboard looking for a chocolate-topped something when the chips are down? Or are we all led down the slippery slope by marketing and advertising, which can make even fatty foods look sexy? Or is it all of the above?

Broadly, we can define factors that have an effect on our food choices and regulation as either internal (or personal factors under the Furst Model, p. 18) such as our taste receptors, emotions, physiology, motivation etc.; or external (contextual factors, for example) such as the food and its components or the environment. Table 2 further explores some of these factors.

Table 2: Factors that influence food intake

Internal	External
Taste physiology such as our sensitivity to salty or sweet tastes	The food itself and its components
Psychology such as our mood and motivation and how this drives us to consume or avoid foods	Environmental factors such as the environment in which we consume the food, and marketing and advertising
Physiological regulators such as hormones that control energy intake or maybe even our genes	Social factors including our socialisation and even who we mix with

In this chapter we will look at both internal and external factors on food choice and regulation. Understanding and acknowledging these factors can be a powerful tool in amending behaviours and attitudes towards food as well as a way of recognising the complexity of food and its effect on us.

Internal factors

Internal factors that affect our taste and food regulation include taste physiology — for example tastebuds and taste sensitivity, plus the hormones involved in hunger and satiety (fullness) — and our internal states such as our personality and mood.

Let's take a look at what happens when we put food in our mouths: our internal taste physiology, how we taste foods, and how this may affect what we choose to eat or not as the case may be.

Taste physiology

Our palate seems able to detect many subtle flavours in our food and drink. However, there are currently only a few distinct taste sensations that we know of. You'll know most of these.

- **Sweet is a reaction that appears to be caused by sugar/s and some proteins and alcohols.**

- **Bitter taste occurs when one or more of the 30 different proteins in our tastebud cells react to bitter chemicals in foods and drinks. Our sensitivity to bitter tastes varies from person to person.**

- **Sour tastes are caused from hydrogen ions in acidic foods and drinks reacting with tastebuds.**

- **Salty, more on this one shortly.**

- **Umami (savoury) is thought to be caused by compounds such as glutamic acid or aspartic acid (amino acids found in foods such as ripe tomatoes, meat, cheese, asparagus) and also added to foods for taste.**

It is quite possible that there are many more tastes that remain undetected, such as alkaline, metallic, spicy and so on.

Just how do tastebuds do their thing?

Most of us have checked out our tongue, commonly to see the damage after gulping down something that was way too hot. While doing so you will have noted the tiny bumps all over your tongue; these are often assumed to be our tastebuds. Well, that's partially right. More accurately we would describe the hundreds of tiny bumps on our tongue as taste papillae. Keep in mind that we also have tastebuds in other areas of the mouth and throat, making the mouth a rich area for taste detection. It's those papillae that have a number of tastebuds within them.

Tastebuds (which look a little like a flower bud, see Figure 2 overleaf) are a group of cells linked together by nerve fibres, which track back to the brain. Each tiny tastebud (of which we have between 2000 and 4000 on our tongue) has up to 50 different cells that are tuned in to various senses. Children up to about the age of ten tend to have many more tastebuds than adults, which might account for the lengthy stage of fussy eating some parents must endure (more on this later). Like skin cells, tastebuds have a pore at the tip which channels down to an inner area where nerve fibres are located. At any nerve junction a multitude of chemicals ebb and flow, creating sensations and electrical impulses that the brain interprets. Like most cells in the body tastebuds are also broken down and replaced; this could be an important factor for altering taste preferences as we will see later.

Figure 2: Tastebud structures[1]

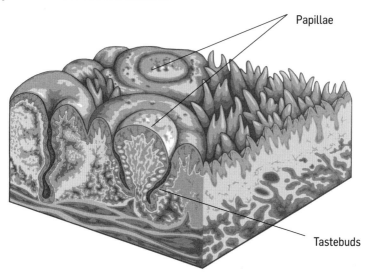

Papillae

Tastebuds

TYPES OF PAPILLAE

Papillae are divided into four basic forms, although filiform papillae don't play a role in taste so won't be discussed here.

Fungiform papillae are the most abundant in our mouth (around 400) and are all over our tongue, but are more dense on the tip of the tongue and around the edges. Not only sensitive to taste, fungiform papillae detect touch and temperature, which probably accounts for why the tip of your tongue is so sensitive.

Circumvallate papillae are larger papillae around the back of our tongue that we can see in the mirror. While we only have a dozen or so of these papillae each one has thousands of tastebuds. As you can see in Figure 3, circumvallate papillae have a moat-like shape where substances can wash over the tastebuds, ensuring a good response.

Foliate papillae are small in number again but being larger are also easy to see. They are found around the back edges of the tongue. Once again, there are hundreds of tastebuds within each of these papillae.

Figure 3: Tastebud receptors on the tongue[2]

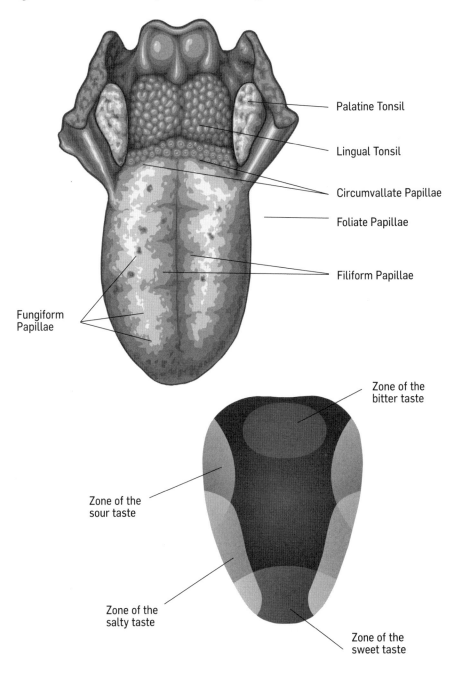

Palatine Tonsil

Lingual Tonsil

Circumvallate Papillae

Foliate Papillae

Filiform Papillae

Fungiform
Papillae

Zone of the
bitter taste

Zone of the
sour taste

Zone of the
salty taste

Zone of the
sweet taste

Fussy eaters and taste sensitivity

It also seems that we experience taste to differing degrees. Our sensitivity to taste (known as taste acuity) affects how we accept new foods. For example, it is likely that some children who are picky eaters have a high taste acuity and are less likely to adjust to new foods, whereas children who have a lowered taste sensitivity respond more favourably to new foods and tastes. It's suggested that children with hypersensitive taste acuity can be predisposed to reject new and novel foods and flavours. Some fussy foodies can be picked out quite easily — they are the ones who 'taste' a food with their lips before allowing the morsel anywhere near their mouth, or sniff a meal before deciding whether it gets the thumbs up. Aha, some of you are saying!

If you are the parent of a fussy eater you will have been advised over and over to offer foods repeatedly to improve acceptance. However, research in the area of food neophobia (fear of novel foods) in children suggests that children with heightened taste sensitivity are less likely to respond to attempts to increase food acceptance by such efforts. But it's not all bad. It seems that at around the ten-year mark the number of tastebuds a child has begins to diminish and often fussy eaters become more willing to try new foods. This is when you begin to finally see all your hard work pay off!

Taste sensations starts early

Our ability to sense taste and smell starts *in utero*, which is probably much earlier than you might think. Prominent researchers in the area of early taste sensation have found that by the third trimester of a pregnancy, a foetus can detect odours of the mother's meals via the amniotic fluid. Foetuses also seem to have early preferences; studies show that a foetus may swallow more amniotic fluid when it is higher in sweet compounds and reduce intake when it is more bitter.[3]

How do specific taste sensations develop?

Let's take a short foray into the world of taste physiology and explore just how taste actually works. Persevere with this as you will find it explains why we prefer some tastes over others and how some tastes appear to have more influence over our food choices than others.

THE PROCESS OF SWEET TASTE SENSATION

To date only a few sweet taste receptors have been discovered (T1R2:T1R3 for the physiologically keen), although there are many receptor sites and likely more receptors will be uncovered. T1R3 along with T1R1 also seems to code for the detection of the umami taste. The preference for sweet tastes seems to be our only innate taste preference; that is, we are born with it rather than it being learnt as a consequence of our environment. We're also designed to reject bitter tastes; some suggest this is a survival mechanism so we don't ingest poison, particularly when we are young and prone to picking up all manner of things and popping them into our mouths. Potentially this could explain why so many children seem to be predisposed to reject all those lovely vegetable-based purées and mashes we start them off with, particularly meals containing vegies that err on the bitter side. While researchers have been able to show an evolutionary influence over food tastes in animals, via breeding rodents that dislike sweet tastes, we humans seem to have something a little more rigorous in place. In fact, it can be quite difficult to influence such innate taste preferences, as we shall see.

Fussy eating in early childhood

So that's why those lovely fruit purées parents offer their babies go down so well, and why somehow baby knows when they are being offered a vegetable and clamps their mouth tightly shut! A variety of healthy foods throughout the solids stage is very important, so keep the balance tilted towards vegies. Parents, be encouraged to continue offering a particular food if baby rejects it; it may just be a matter of time before baby's tastebuds adapt to the more bitter foods. While the preference for sweet tastes is one given by nature, we as parents still control the environment: remember, 'parents offer, children choose'. If we give in to the sweet tastes it gets harder to amend this; keeping home for the good stuff and leaving the sweet stuff for outings can also help.

Our preference for sweet-tasting foods, however, seems to be multifactorial, being influenced possibly by genetics (although the jury is still out on this one), social influences and our environment, including exposure and our own physiology. There is some research suggesting other physiological factors, such as glucose transporters (mechanisms for the digestion and absorption of glucose — or GLUT2 for those of you wanting more technical information), may somehow play a role in some individuals' preferences for sweet foods. Put more simply, some of the mechanisms involved in glucose absorption appear to have more influence on the preference for sweet foods than sweet taste receptors do.

Non-nutritive sweeteners:
Is the deception worth it?

Are you one of the many people who opt for the 'zero' sugars products, ones that use artificial sweeteners (referred to as non-nutritive sweeteners)? Ever wondered how they do their thing?

Once in our mouths, the sugars found naturally in our diet may well prime our digestive system for digestion. Technically, our palate responds to food by beginning something referred to as the pre-absorptive metabolic phase of digestion.

While we have adapted to respond to non-nutritive sweeteners (just how is not yet clear), it seems even without calories they promote the gaining of excess weight by interfering with pre-absorptive processes when we eat food. In most cases, natural unadulterated options are better for health.

ARE YOU A BITTER SUPERTASTER?

Many suggest that sensitivity to bitter tastes has a survival component to it, in that recognising bitter tastes may prevent us from consuming poisonous plants and foods. If we look back over the literature from early last century onwards regarding our sensitivity to bitter tastes, people were broadly classified as either 'tasters' or 'non-tasters' (the latter group being those with less sensitivity to bitter tastes). Just how sensitive you are also may depend on where you come from: people from different regions differ in the ratio of tasters to non-tasters. For example, around 3 per cent of people in West Africa appear to be non-tasters, while up to 23 per cent in China fell into this category and up to as many as 30 per cent in North American Caucasian populations. What's more, 'tasters' can be subdivided into 'medium tasters' and 'supertasters'. Just what accounts for such differences is not yet entirely clear, however, genes appear to play an important role in the expression of tastes such as bitter. For those of you wanting to delve deeper into the workings of bitter taste sensation you will need to look at protein-coupled receptors, called T2Rs, which appear to be controlled by around 25 genes found on chromosomes 5, 7 and 12.[4]

SOUR TASTE PERCEPTION

As soon as you hear or read the word sour you probably think of a raw lemon, and your mouth is probably watering even now. The process of sour taste perception involves chemical interactions. Simply put, when our tastebuds come into contact with acidic substances this causes a chemical reaction (known as depolarisation) that allows chemicals such as calcium to pass into the tastebud receptor cells, beginning a chain reaction which ultimately leads to a taste sensation. Because many acid compounds — such as acetic, citric, lactic and tartaric acids

— are found in fermenting products it's been suggested that, like bitter tastes, the detection of sour may also perform a survival function. Detecting sour can prevent us from eating unripe fruit or food that is spoilt and off (which is undergoing fermentation — remember the last time you drank fermented milk?).

In reality, not much more is known about sour taste. There are lots of theories, but to date there's very little hard evidence about what causes sour taste perception and why it can differ so widely between people.

SALT TASTE PERCEPTION

You would think that given the degree to which salt plays a part in our eating that we would know a whole lot about it, but no. Just how salt taste perception occurs is, believe it or not, unclear. Salt channels (sodium chloride, NaCl, to be precise) in fungiform papillae appear to be responsible, at least in part, for salt taste perception. Given our present knowledge the idea of genetic influence doesn't have a great deal of support (though this theory could change with more research). Sensitivity to salty tastes varies widely from one person to another, and it appears that it's our environment that has the greatest impact on salt taste sensitivity. If we consider studies on twins (used because of their genetic similarity) in the area of salt taste sensitivity, it appears twins' sensitivity is similar more as a result of their eating habits (environment) than their genetics.

Salt is an interesting compound. It predominates our foods and many people just can't get enough; most of us know at least one person who adds salt to every meal, even ones that are already salted. So we're going to take a much closer look at our love of salt shortly when we look at food preferences. For now, we are just taking a brief look at physiological influences on salt taste perception.

UMAMI: SAVOURING YOUR FOOD

Umami is a Japanese derived word for 'good taste' and relates to our detection of savoury flavours. Umami is detected in response to an amino acid in many foods, called L-glutamate and occurring as monosodium glutamate (yes, the stuff that used to be added to many Asian dishes). If you've ever had any experience with monosodium glutamate (MSG as it's commonly known) you would be forgiven for thinking it was a salt-based product. Umami can often be confused for salty tastes but, in fact, being a savoury taste it is quite different. Not a great deal is known about how umami taste detection works, though as mentioned before it seems closely aligned to sweet taste detection simply because these receptors are also sensitive to L-glutamate.

WHAT ABOUT FAT?

Fat is the stuff that makes food taste not just good but in some cases *really* good! It's widely known that we seem to have a knack for picking out foods that contain fat. Hence, fat taste perception was initially believed to be more about texture than taste. But there appears to be more to this story than meets the eye. What would you expect when it comes to the nutrient that provides us with more energy per gram than any other?

We now know that fat detection is about more than texture; studies show that if fat texture is inhibited our uncanny knack to find the fat is unaffected. Clearly, there is more to fat taste detection than just the physical properties of fat.

Currently it's thought we have at least one fat receptor on our tongue, which would make 'fatty' the sixth taste perception. It seems we have a receptor (or receptors) that respond to saturated fatty acids, such as oleic and stearic fatty acids, plus unsaturated fatty acids, such as linoleic acid (see Table 3), and it is possible there are other receptors for other fatty acids. Receptors such as Fatty Acid Transporter (FAT), G-protein receptors (GPR) that use fatty acids (smallest components of the fat we eat) and fatty acid receptor CD36 have been detected in the circumvallate and foliate papillae of the tongue. It appears, though, that the signals are more of a contextual nature, relating to the texture of fat as opposed to the taste.[5]

Research into the specific receptors, mechanism and genes responsible for fatty taste sensitivity is still in its infancy and there's a great deal to uncover in this area of taste. Given that we seem predisposed to seek out fatty foods and many countries are experiencing weight control issues, the area of fat perception has something to it, though the influence of fat intake on weight may turn up some surprising findings.

UPDATE ON OUR KNOWLEDGE OF SATURATED FAT AND HEALTH
Hold on to your hat! Most of us will be familiar with the catchphrase 'unsaturated fat good, saturated fat bad'. It seems that we have been a little misled. Researchers have recently found that not all saturated fatty acids (each class of fat has a number of different types of fatty acids in it) are bad for us. Saturated fats with carbon chains between 12 and 16 increase cholesterol, whereas those over 18 don't seem to cause the same health issues — stearic acid and oleic acid, for example. (Take a look at Table 3 for some examples of the kinds of foods containing saturated fatty acids, along with the carbon chain length for each.) It appears that myristic acid, followed by lauric acid and palmitic acid are the 'less desirable' fats. Some foods contain a number of different types of saturated fatty acids, for example butter, which further complicates our understanding of what constitutes a 'healthy' food.

So for us everyday mortals this might suggest that trying to understand all the science can just make the task of eating well harder, and that perhaps just focusing on a variety of healthy whole foods is the way to go.

Table 3: Saturated fatty acid sources

Name	Length of carbon chain	Food sources
Arachidic acid (eicosanoic)	20	Peanuts
Stearic acid** (octodecanoic)	18	Beef, mutton, pork, butter, cocoa butter (i.e. dark chocolate)
Palmitic acid* (hexadecanoic)	16	Tropical fats such as coconut, palm and palm kernel
Myristic acid* (tetradecanoic)	14	Coconut oil and butter
Lauric acid* (dodecanoic)	12	Coconut oil
Caprioc acid (hexanoic)	6	Dairy fat
Buytyric acid (butanoic)	4	Dairy, e.g. butter

*Found to raise plasma lipoprotein fractions
**No effect on plasma lipoproteins

Taste physiology in perspective

Conscious or mindful eating may well be a central factor in our health. Just like so many things we do almost automatically, eating, too, may be best brought into a more conscious realm. Have you ever jumped in the car and driven off, without a thought, then suddenly got to a point and realised you'd driven to the wrong destination? Given then that our taste physiology is in part under our control and in part unconscious, surely the more aware we are of this the more healthful our eating, and potentially our lifestyle, will be. We'll look more at this concept throughout the book. Conscious eating, remember that!

Let's now take a look at the physiological processes that control our food intake.

FOOD INTAKE REGULATION

The factors causing us to eat more or less, and that cause us to stop eating and feel full, are varied and being discovered and revised with great fervour. Physiological factors, in particular, are of great interest since the realisation that so many of us are ballooning and that, despite great efforts, the trend is proving difficult to reverse. You have to wonder about the benefit of attributing overeating to our hormones and chemicals — and the 'chicken or the egg argument' rears its head in this regard from time to time; nonetheless we must concede that a host of hormones, receptors and chemicals appear to be involved in our food intake regulation.

A cascade of events leads from feeling hungry, to eating and then satiety (feeling full). Each step in the cascade involves myriad biochemical and physiological processes that are beyond the scope of this book. However, it's helpful to have under our belt a basic understanding of how we progress from being hungry to feeling full, and there are a plethora of terms with which we should be at least vaguely familiar before we move forward. The cascade of events in the process of food intake regulation is briefly as follows (internal regulation fills in the gaps).

- **HUNGER is the drive to fulfil a physiological need for survival. This is our basic drive; in other words we eat to survive.**

- **APPETITE, our desire to eat, is stimulated by physiological states and/or by food via sensory signals (for example, suddenly feeling hungry when you smell food).**

- **FOOD is ingested; that is, it's eaten.**

- **SATIATION (or the act of creating satiety) causes you to stop eating.**

- **SATIETY (that lovely sense of feeling full) occurs when two things happen: our sensory and cognitive (thinking) states begin to inhibit hunger and appetite; and post-ingestive and post-absorptive hormones are secreted during satiety (in other words, hormones start to kick into action very early on, even before we start eating until long after we have finished our meal).**

Body wisdom

Some findings suggest that while animals have excellent 'body wisdom' and are innately able to maintain internal 'balance' (a state known as homoeostasis), we humans are not so adept. Up until around the age of two we are very good at self-regulating our energy intake. That's why it's important to honour young children's eating cues (rather than, for example, asking them to finish their meal simply to please us or to eat because it's a certain time of day) or we risk overriding their self-regulation, the result being a loss of touch with internal cues of hunger and fullness. This may well help explain why we can be so susceptible to 'portion distortion'.

The weight-loss industry is already tapping into the myriad factors involved in our food regulation, as seen in the increasing array of weight-loss products such as those using bulking agents, which act to stimulate stretch receptors in the gut and create a feeling of satiety. While detail can be useful, it is worth remembering that, at times, detail can obscure some of the most simple and influential factors. We will take a good look at our awareness of hunger and satiety body cues soon, and as we will see, they are simple but effective internal cues which many with weight issues have ignored for too long.

The flow from hunger to satiety is not always quite this simple or logical, however. More specific physiological controls involve areas of the brain including the hypothalamus, where it is suggested a form of 'switch' exists that controls our body weight, making long-term weight-loss extremely challenging for some of us. The hypothalamus secretes protein-based peptides that switch on hunger and encourage us to eat more. More on this later.

Our body secretes a number of substances that affect our hunger and satiety. The hormone cholecystokinin (CCK) is secreted when we eat foods containing fat and protein. CCK assists the breakdown of fat by stimulating the gallbladder (which stores bile, our fat 'detergent') and the pancreas, causing the flow of food from the stomach to the intestines to slow, thereby inhibiting hunger. Then there's leptin, produced in our fat cells, which has become a common word in weight-loss circles. Oxyntomodulin made in our large intestines also plays a role, as do many more substances.

Most of the known substances appear to inhibit hunger, but one, ghrelin, stimulates our hunger. The following excerpt is from a journal article by a presenter at an Australian Scientific Meeting in 2010. It might offer you some insight into the area of food regulation and the numerous compounds that appear to be involved (there's a bit of technical jargon but it makes sense of why diets are so hard to stick to).

Following weight loss, many changes occur that are designed to encourage weight regain. Firstly there is a mild decrease in energy expenditure (maximally about 300 Kcal per day). Ghrelin levels increase while leptin, CCK, insulin, amylin, PYY all decrease. The net effect is for hunger to increase. The weight-reduced obese individual is then in the difficult

situation of being hungrier than normal while being surrounded by freely available food. It is not surprising then that gradual weight regain is almost inevitable.[6]

What the author is suggesting is that when you do finally begin to lose weight your body may be conspiring against you to try to return to your original weight. There are also many other factors that make permanent weight loss a challenge, including our ability to inhibit habits, our personality and so on; but it's interesting to see the extent to which our bodies exert control over our food intake and hunger.

Tip: What healthy eating, which is health focused and not 'diet' focused, will do in part is reshape our headspace and behaviour towards food and eating, permanently.

We should be reminded of the effort we need to put into eating consciously; this includes recognising that changing your body weight for health will be a challenge.

YOUR BRAIN AND HUNGER

The area of neurological control of eating can be a little clinical, possibly because in reality we still don't understand just how it all works, so we'll work up from the basics and give you a taste (excuse the pun) for some of the more complex.

Hunger control is deeply rooted in the neurological circuitry of our brain, specifically in an area called the hypothalamus, though it is likely there are a number of other regions given the diverse factors involved in appetite, hunger and satiation (see Figure 4 on p. 58). Certainly it seems our hypothalamus is more involved in the control of and response to hunger than satiety. What's more, both our physiology and environment (including the food itself) affect our brain differently. Monitoring the brain we can see changes in areas of activation as we move from being hungry to feeling full, but how and why this happens is not yet clear.

Figure 4: The hypothalamus[7]

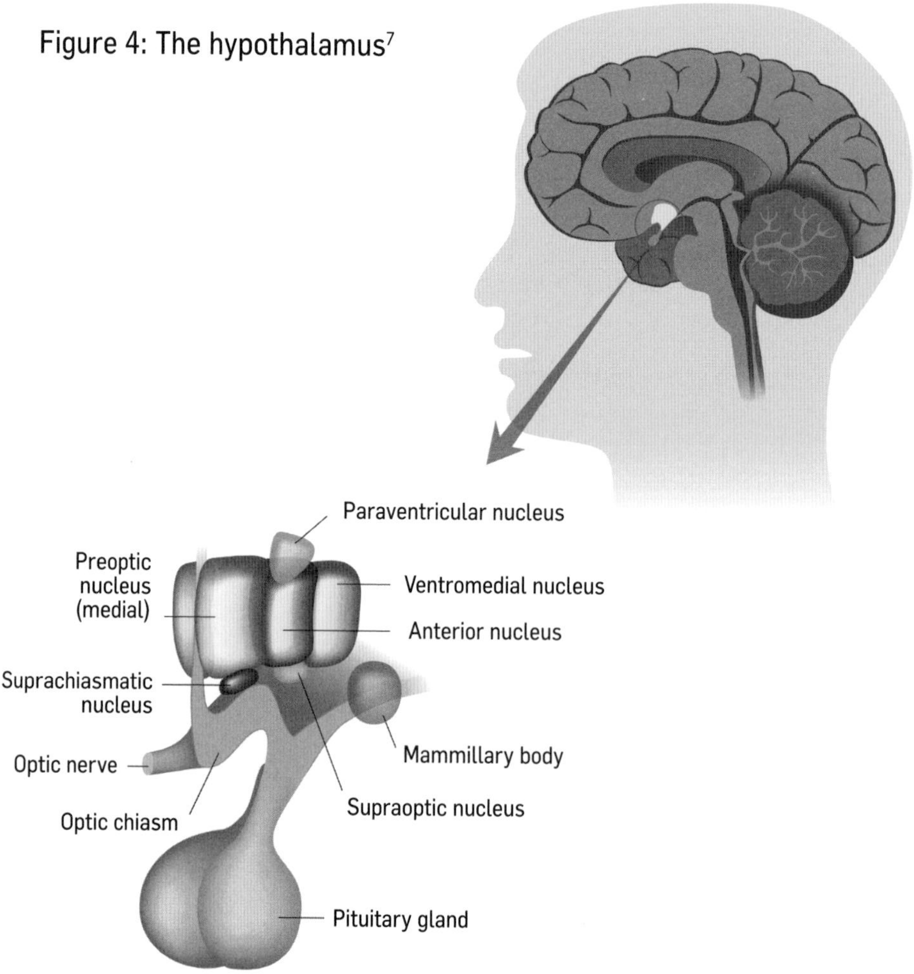

Paraventricular nucleus

Preoptic nucleus (medial)

Ventromedial nucleus

Anterior nucleus

Suprachiasmatic nucleus

Optic nerve

Mammillary body

Optic chiasm

Supraoptic nucleus

Pituitary gland

The parts of the brain involved in our motivation to eat are quite complex and are more of a network of interrelated areas extending from the mid-region of our brain (referred to as the midbrain) through to the outer areas (cortex). Study in this area has led to some great advances in the field of disordered eating (including both under- and overeating). Logically, any dysfunction, damage or imbalance in the neurons in these areas will impact on our desire to eat, how much we eat and how efficient we are at stopping eating. Studies are being conducted on how these areas are turned on and off, what influences them and how they might explain disordered eating and issues of obesity.

That the brain is implicated in the rate of obesity raises questions. For example, does this suggest that we are experiencing more neuronal dysfunction which has led to an increased incidence of obesity compared to the past? If so, what factors have led to this? Is it possible that our 'method' of eating (both how and what we eat) has affected our brain chemistry in some way? You can see how this might be a can of worms!

The pleasure of food

Let's now take a look at how the pleasure of eating works both for and against us. It's thought that the part of our brain considered our 'pleasure centre', referred to as the ventral tegmental area, is involved in hunger. It's further thought that this area holds hedonic pathways (hedonic relating to things we do that give us pleasure) that are involved in the motivation we gain from the reward of food. To put it simply, our brain has pathways that are involved in the pleasure we derive from eating. In fact, the pleasure we gain from food may be so strong that it can override some of our physiological satiety signals, which in turn can be responsible for us eating way more than we should or need.

Something we will look at shortly is just why fat has such a hold over us. One of the keys to this is 'palatability', which sounds a simple term; logically one would assume it refers to how appealing a food or meal is. But it is far more complex than that. Palatability of a food relates more to the hedonic or pleasurable experience a food or a nutrient such as fat creates within us. The level of pleasure we gain from a food will depend on many things, including internal factors such as our brain chemistry (specifically opioid levels), and external factors such as who you are eating with, the atmosphere, the reason you are eating and so on. Now there's a bit more to this palatability caper: it appears that it can also be learnt, hence with repeated behaviours we can literally teach or rewire our brains to enjoy certain foods.

FOOD CRAVINGS

By now you are probably beginning to get a real sense of just how complex hunger and satiety really is and how 'new kids on the block' findings can arrive and completely alter all that we thought we knew. The palatability of food appears to interfere with our physiological satiety signals and yes, you guessed, it causes us to overeat. For example, those added sugars (sucrose or table sugar for example) we consume most commonly from manufactured foods may alter our brain activity by influencing substances that transmit information along neural pathways. This causes an 'overstimulation', which influences pleasure and reward pathways — and results in overeating. This brings us to the area of 'food cravings'. It's believed that these overstimulated pathways cause food cravings, hence cravings are often seen as being embedded in our brains. It's also thought that 'emotional eating' is a result of increased cortisol secretion (commonly secreted during stress), which interferes with dopamine, leading to eating to soothe. All in all, this might explain why we can easily overeat indulgent foods — another argument for conscious eating and the reshaping of our eating habits.

External influences

Let's move to external factors that influence food choice and intake. It's likely you will find this a little revealing or close to the bone, but go with it — some suggest our greatest strength is our vulnerability, so being 'naked' for a while might just do us some good!

We'll look at both food preferences and taste preferences. What is taste preference? Remember we mentioned earlier those who add salt to every meal? That's a taste preference. Simply put, taste preference describes why we choose one taste over another (for example, sweet over savoury), while food preference, or choice, describes why we choose one food over another (for example, steak instead of chicken).

Food preferences

There are a range of things that influence our choices of food. They include our ability to:

- **learn**
- **recall/remember**
- **make decisions**
- **interact with others.**

Food choice is influenced as we know by many internal (biological/physiological and psychological) factors. These choices are believed to be further influenced by three main external factors:

- **EXPOSURE**, for example when we are exposed to certain ways of eating through cultural habits and family practices.

- **CLASSICAL LEARNING**, for example associating a food with a certain taste or behaviour. Many parents avoid sugar as they believe it makes their usually calm child overactive, and hence associate sugar with hyperactivity. (This is not actually the case; it's more likely the fault of the additives that tend to accompany sugary foods.)

- **SOCIAL LEARNING**, as is the case of peer learning, for example when your teenager comes home a newly formed vegetarian and upon questioning you find out it's more because 'everyone is doing it' rather than for any philosophical or nutritional reason.

Your preference for savoury foods over sweet will likely, at least in part, be a learnt preference. So too is a child's preference for white foods — yes, those fussy foodies who will only eat pasta, white rice, fries and chicken nuggets. We need to be mindful of the many factors that have influenced our food choices and eating habits; some of these were explored when we discussed the Furst Model of Food Choice (p. 18), so if you need to reconsider your learnt choices and habits review this section.

SOCIAL FACILITATION

Ever heard of social facilitation? In a nutshell it's all about the influences around us that encourage eating. Simple things such as music, heating, lighting, who we eat with, how many people are eating with us and so on. The influence of social facilitation on eating has been well researched. You won't be surprised to learn that myriad factors influence what we eat and how much. Here are just a few examples.

- When alone we tend to eat fewer meals and with less energy (calories). This can be a common issue as we get older and the nest empties, which is tricky simply because as we age we need fewer calories but often more nutrients.

- If we throw a bit of alcohol into the mix with a meal, we tend to consume (yes, you guessed it) more food.

- As the saying goes, the more the merrier. The same goes for eating — the more friends we have with us at a meal the longer we tend to sit and the more we eat and drink.

- Notice that in most places where food is accompanied by background music, it tends to be slower music. That's largely because we tend to hang about longer when slow music is being played, for example in restaurants, and not only do we eat more but — much to the delight of the manager — we drink more too.

- We also tend to eat more when we believe we are eating in a quality establishment. For example, we might eat a little more when in a 4-star restaurant as opposed to a café.

Most of us will relate to these events, and of course we can do our best to moderate them if we need to. In most cases a social setting is just that: a setting where we go to be with others, often outside of our own home.

The effects of social factors can extend beyond overeating; they also have implications for children who are fussy eaters, people with disordered eating and those who require increased nourishment, such as isolated elderly people. For example:

- **Seating a good eater with a fussy eater can increase the chances of the once good eater picking up some fussy habits.**

- **Seating a picky eater next to a peer who models good eating actually has greater impact than if you seat the picky eater next to a teacher who models good eating.**

- **Elderly people living alone are at greater risk of undernourishment simply from not being motivated to cook for themselves.**

We also know that recommendations by waiters or other people significantly influence our food choices, both positively and negatively depending on the positive or negative recommendation respectively. So if you own a restaurant, the way your staff runs through the meals of the day or answers questions on recommendations can have a strong impact on which dishes are popular. But before you stop asking for recommendations, or rush out and retrain your staff, keep in mind that while these factors exert some degree of influence they don't exert as much influence over our hedonic response to the food once we have consumed it. In other words, we make up our own mind when tasting a food, so the recommendation and the experience had better match up.

LIKING AND WANTING ARE DIFFERENT

We should also keep in mind that *liking* and *wanting* are two different things. I can like sugar but after my eighth sweet I might not want any more. It also seems that liking is easier to affect and influence, while wanting seems more deeply 'ingrained' within us and less susceptible to change.

Liking relates to the pleasure we derive from eating (called oro-sensory stimulation to be precise). It's believed to be influenced by opiate systems in our brain. Studies in animals have shown that it's possible to inhibit liking and wanting separately via neural pathways in the brain. Hence *wanting* is a motivational state, one that drives us to eat, and thought to be influenced by dopaminergic brain systems.

Liking activates food choice or preference, which determines what is eaten (though there can be many factors that influence this process).

A sweet tooth

It is commonly believed that overweight people have a 'sweet tooth', a preference for sweet foods. However, research suggests that overweight individuals have no greater liking of sweet foods than normal weight individuals. In fact, it appears that motivation is a more salient factor in obesity, with obese individuals being more motivated just generally by food itself.

When do taste preferences start?

You often hear people saying our early years are an important time for setting up healthy eating habits; but you might be surprised to learn just how early taste preferences can begin.

Research has shown that taste preferences develop as early as the foetal stage. Studies have demonstrated if a mother eats a certain food while pregnant (for example, carrots), then her baby will be more accepting of the food when they begin solids. The same effect occurs via breastmilk. What's more, this early exposure for baby leads to a wider array of tastes and may increase acceptance of foods down the track. Keep in mind that just because an expectant mother does not eat a particular food doesn't necessarily mean their bub will not eat or enjoy that food later.

Let's take a look at some of the common taste preferences; we all have someone in the family who loves salty food, or craves fatty food, or can't say no to sweets.

PREFERENCE FOR SALTY FOODS

A liking for salty (and fatty) foods is something that we learn. Neonatal studies show that newborns can't tell the difference between varying intensity of salt solutions; on this basis, salt preference is said to be a learnt taste preference. Sensitivity, or our ability to detect salty solution, appears to kick off around four months of age, but from here on it's all about our environment exerting considerable influence over our great fondness for salty tastes. Our preference for salty taste increases over our first year and with great consistency for us all. It is a sustained exposure to salt that leads us to be very 'loyal' to its use and our preference for salty foods in adulthood. Of course, we are all different and in fact it is our individual sensitivity to salt that appears to ultimately influence just how much we like salt and seek out excessively salty foods.

We have already been introduced to 'supertasters' who have increased taste papillae. Salt supertasters report a greater sensitivity to salt solutions — simply put, they can detect salt much faster than the rest of it is. If you're a supertaster you'll notice more changes in taste sensation when salt is added to food, but you'll also have an increased liking for that food, which will lead you to eat even more of it.

The good news is that as we reduce our use of sodium our

sensitivity is lowered; so all we need to do to adjust to this new taste sensation of less salt is just use less. However, we need to keep in mind that some studies have found that altering sensitisation might influence our *wanting* of salt but not our *liking*; in other words, for some of us cutting back on salt might reduce our desire to have it so frequently but do nothing for our love of the stuff when confronted with it.

CHILDREN AND SALTY FOOD

It's important to keep in mind that our environment exerts considerable control over our love of salty (and fatty) foods. Don't let the horse bolt, that's the key! As we will see, food habits formed during early childhood appear to be the hardest to change. Avoid using salt in children's meals and remember most of our salt comes from processed foods (80 per cent). Children who are exposed to salt early on and repeatedly ingest it are very likely going to grow into adults who love their salt.

Tip: The good news is that everyone can adjust to less salt and less salty-tasting foods. Simply slowly reducing the salt, opting for low-salt foods and avoiding heavily salted products will quickly result in a readjustment of your tastebuds. Before you know it you can detect all sorts of fabulous tastes and you will baulk at an overly salted meal.

Healthful eating task:
Reducing your salt intake

Cutting back on salt and trying to reshape your want for salty foods can be a worthy exercise given most of the salt in our diet comes from pre-prepared, pre-packaged or processed foods which can tend to be on the 'unhealthy options' side of the menu.

Select some of the strategies below that resonate with you. Put them into action along with avoiding using salt at home, and you'll find that you will be eating healthier.

- **Chose to move to 'salt-reduced' options for foods notoriously high in salt, including sauces, chips (crisps), soups, spreads and cheese.**

- **Opt for sourdough or unleavened breads (it's the self-raising flour with bicarbonate of soda (baking soda) that significantly increases the sodium content).**

- **Cut back on canned foods, perhaps using them only once a week or reduce by one per week.**

- **Cut back on cured meats (ham, bacon, salami) and opt for canned fish in springwater etc. instead.**

- **Cut down on the number of takeaway meals you eat (restaurants and fast food places serve heavily salted meals).**

- **Drink water instead of sports drinks when you are not exercising.**

Our preference for fatty foods

Fat really is in a league of its own! Our preference for fatty foods appears to be learnt in a similar fashion to salt, however, our ability to detect and react to fat levels in food is quite different. And while we are able to adjust to a diet lower in fatty tastes, it seems we find it much harder to stick to such diets. While our taste perceptions can adjust, our want and love for fatty foods lags behind. Many dieters will attest to this.

It may take some time before our love of fat is reshaped sufficiently for us to make a permanent change in our eating habits, and for it to be one that we truly enjoy. This might explain why, after we have enjoyed a diet rich in fatty foods we find healthy food a little on the 'dim' side tastewise in the early days. As we will see soon, one of the keys to successfully changing your eating habits is a sustained effort focused on small changes; the longer you stick at it the less you will be tempted away and the more likely the change will be permanent. Also keep in mind that fat is not necessarily the bad guy as we once thought. Demonising a nutrient may serve to only be a distraction from the changes we need to make in reshaping our own eating habits and choices.

Tip: **Being fearful of food is not helpful — we should be able to enjoy all foods, eating relevant amounts of them without guilt but from a mindful and conscious health perspective.**

Hunger is not a friend of healthy eating. Hunger prevents us from making good eating choices and this is true in respect to fat. Our love of fatty foods is heightened when we are hungry, and possibly this is due to the density of energy fat contains — that is, it's a food that can quickly add to our energy coffers. How many of us haven't felt that urge for a greasy takeaway after a long day without food? Hunger is not our friend when we are trying to make good food choices! So hunger and time go hand in hand: most of us have about three to four hours of stored energy in our muscle and liver, so we can go comfortably for that long between meals (depending on our bodies and activity amongst other things). We don't need to eat all day, but rather should have good healthy eating patterns to prevent hunger leading us astray.

As mentioned earlier, researchers now believe we have at least one fat receptor in our mouth, but just what role such receptors have in taste preference is not yet clear; they may release endorphins and dopamine (involved in our sense of wellbeing) or cause satiety. However, given fat itself doesn't fill us up (it has a low satiety effect) and hence doesn't cause satiation (cessation of eating) you have to wonder just where fat gets its powers from. Potentially, the lack of physical effects that fat creates may be overcome by the psychological affects it appears to be able to provoke within us.

The influence of 'good tasting food'

Let's return to the influence of palatability, the hedonic or pleasurable experience that a food or a nutrient such as fat creates within us. The level of pleasure we get from a food will depend on many things, including our brain chemistry (specifically opioid levels), who we are eating with, the atmosphere, the reason we are eating and so on. We have discovered that palatability can be learnt, but is strong enough to override our natural cues of hunger and satiety (fullness). That's why you can so very easily overeat indulgent foods.

Can you guess when the palatability of a particular food is greatest? Yes, when we are deprived of that food; and palatability is at its lowest just after we have eaten it. This makes perfect sense of all those times you give in to a dessert you're craving but afterwards you suddenly feel the anticipation was better than the experience. Still we do this time and time again, which brings us back to liking and wanting being quite different things. While you can reduce your liking of something, the wanting still remains a salient factor. Research seems to suggest that our wanting of a food is not easily controlled because it may be governed by processes beyond our mere physiology. Just how this works is not as yet understood, though it is likely that our higher order processes (such as our emotions) are involved.

Sticking with the idea that palatability of foods can be learnt, it's believed some of us learn 'hedonic hunger' — a hunger that is not just physiological but psychological — a hunger that is beyond or overrides the body's natural self-regulating systems. In essence this might put into question the role of food manufacturers in the weight issues of so many countries. Perhaps mere public education alone is in some cases insufficient to stem the tide; maybe we also need to look more closely at the quality of food being amassed on our shelves and in stores. Surely, if food can have such a strong hold over us there needs to be more invested into the quality production of food that is on offer.

The importance of body cues

When the evidence on the effectiveness of weight-loss strategies is reviewed, it appears that:

- **dieting is by and large ineffective over the long term but effective for short-term weight loss**
- **dieting can have a significant negative impact psychologically**

- non-dieting approaches don't appear to provide significant weight loss but over the long term they are more sustainable
- non-dieting tends to have a positive psychological impact.

And if you are daring you might suggest that what all this says is that the key to a healthy body weight is healthy eating habits.

Habits! We'll look at this more closely soon, but for now let's focus on behaviour and learning. It is highly likely that what is needed is reshaping of behaviours. This reshaping needs to override old limiting and unhealthy behaviours and reform with new healthful behaviours and choices. This takes time; a slow and steady approach is needed in order to create new ways of interpreting and reacting, to the point where the new behaviours become second nature. So our old autopilot love of fatty foods becomes overridden with a new, unconscious enjoyment of fresh foods; in fact, this is where we started at birth. If you are thinking 'that sounds way too hard', don't be put off.

Tip: Eating well is innate for all healthy beings; unhealthy eating is something we adapt to. We have overridden the innate neural pathways of healthful eating with self-defeating habits — we simply need to rewrite, reshape if you like, or reform habits and return to where we started.

Research and even anecdotal evidence shows us that the current paradigm of 'dieting' is:

- difficult to maintain in the long term
- yields reasonably low positive outcomes and doesn't appear to have significantly interrupted the overweight figures
- can end in harmful outcomes related to poor self-esteem, poor body image and negative emotional states.

A new view of weight issues focuses instead not on weight loss but on health. The Health at Every Size (HAES) approach, a term first coined by Linda Bacon, promotes altering our eating habits in relation to increasing our health. HAES supports an acceptance of the natural variation of body shapes and sizes, and studies using this method appear to show greatly improved outcomes to the dieting approach, including:

- improvement in psychological issues of depression, body image and self-esteem
- reshaped eating habits with less susceptibility to hunger and habitual eating.[8]

By using health-centred approaches to eating we may well be able to reshape the eating habits that cause us grief. By improving our ability to detect and respond to our own internal cues of hunger and fullness we can improve our health. Now this is not to say that we have to think about every single meal from here on in. What will happen is, as we relearn how we interact with food, we will create new pathways in our brain and what we once had to consciously consider will become second nature. You will be inclined to eat healthier foods, be less swayed by unhealthy options, unconsciously make healthier choices and actually enjoy food. You will even know when you can have 'treats' and won't need to beat yourself up or counter the treat with a punishment.

People who struggle with weight issues often find it difficult to restrain themselves. They can eat enormous amounts despite being full and it's not until afterwards that they realise they have overeaten, often winding up with great guilt and sometimes shame. But if you compare them to 'normal weight' individuals such thoughts of restraint and even issues of temptation simply aren't present. This is where we are heading: towards a normalised eating for health.

Naturally, this isn't likely to happen overnight, and we will look closely at how habits are formed and changed. The overall message is to be realistic — slow and steady wins the race.

The following table shows you a range of hunger and fullness levels. If you read over this you will note that you have at some time in your life experienced each, but as we get older many of us stop listening to these cues.

We'll come back to these ranges shortly when we look at using them to reshape our eating habits.

Table 4: Levels of hunger and satiety

Too hungry	'I feel as if I could be sick.'
	'I feel light-headed, shaky and fuzzy.'
Hunger aware	'My stomach is gurgling from hunger pains.'
	'I really need something in my stomach and can't stop thinking about food.'
Neutral	'I'm not really hungry but don't feel satisfied.'
	'I don't feel hungry.'
Satisfied fullness	'I'm starting to feel full and have stopped eating.'
	'I feel nicely full.'
Excessively full	'I really need to loosen my belt and feel too full.'
	'I have eaten way too much and feel very uncomfortable and sickly.'

What do hunger and fullness feel like?

The reality is these are terms that can be quite specific for each of us. While most of us would associate hunger with feelings ranging from a growling stomach, pains in the stomach through to feeling nauseated and dizzy, it's best to use your own rating. Next time you eat consider how you feel about two to three hours later. Most of us have enough stored body energy to last us about three hours comfortably but by four hours we are getting really hungry.

Tip: It takes roughly twenty minutes for the process of satiety to occur. In other words, it takes twenty minutes from the time you start eating to the time your body signals to your brain that you are full. Avoid judging your level of fullness or hunger within twenty minutes of a meal; if you wonder just ten minutes after your first helping whether you need more, the answer will likely be a resounding 'yes'.

Healthful eating task: Create your own hunger and fullness scale

Using Table 4 as a guide, create your own self-rating scale so you can become more aware of how long it takes to become noticeably hungry, how long before you begin to be uncomfortable, or when you can't take your mind of food, through to when you begin to exhibit actual signs of hunger such as hunger pangs or nausea.

Also become aware of what it feels like to be comfortably full and then consider how it feels to be overfull. Perhaps this includes ranging from feeling as if your abdomen is so stretched you need to loosen your pants, to feeling as if your stomach is so full it could almost make its way back up your oesophagus.

Get to know your body cues and use them

Now that you're becoming familiar with body cues it's time to really get in touch with your own body. Do the following exercise for three weeks, on six out of every seven days. Try to rate your level of desire to eat a meal, the level of hunger you feel, the amount you believe you will eat, and then the level of fullness that results. Make three photocopies of Table 5 on p. 78 to monitor your findings, then write down your answers for each day.

Table 5: Self-monitoring

Day	How strong is your desire to eat? (Choose: none, mild, or extreme)			How hungry do you feel? (Choose: not at all, mildly, or extremely)			How much food do you think you need to eat? (Choose: none, some, or a lot)			Rate how you feel 20 minutes after a meal (Choose: nothing, perfect, or overfull)		
1												
2												
3												
4												
5												
6												
Day off												

Remember, waiting twenty minutes will allow all your body signals to develop so you will be better able to decide if you are still hungry or not. Don't be tempted to eat one helping straight after another.

When we look at habits shortly you will be able to expand on this activity by including behavioural strategies to help you reach your goals. Together, increasing your body awareness as well as using strategies to reduce temptation will make it so much easier to stay on track.

How food affects what and how much we eat

So, can the food itself affect our eating? The simple answer is yes. For example, we know now that nutrients such as protein help our bodies to switch to 'full' mode and stop us eating. Many people refer to protein as the 'satiety' nutrient. In fact, it seems that protein has a stronger satiety effect than carbohydrate and much more than fat. Ah, you say, that makes sense of why you can eat a load of fatty burgers and still feel hungry. It might also make sense of why we see so much about high protein diets and weight loss. Remember, you can have too much of a good thing — balance is essential! When you tip the nutritional scales in favour of one nutrient or compound it can put other areas out of balance. Studies show that some amino acids (small units of protein) have different levels of satiety, so clearly it's not straightforward, particularly as our knowledge expands. The main message is: ensure you consume a variety of protein-containing foods throughout the day to help you feel less hungry. So often we eat snacks such as fruit, which is great, but without the protein they can leave you prey to hunger! Try adding a little protein to the mix, like a small tub of natural yoghurt.

Tip: **Hunger and bad food choices are 'joined at the hip', so avoiding hunger while still being tuned into your body signals will go a long way in helping you stick with healthy eating options.**

Just the presence of food itself appears to will some of us to eat it. For example, it seems that, in some cases, those of us who are overweight are more attentive to food in our environment than non-overweight people. This is even more so when hunger is a factor. Remember, hunger is not our friend when we are trying to alter body weight. Let's put this into context. There you are happily swigging down your apparently satiating meal substitute, a shake all padded out with fibre, in the hope it'll make you feel full and therefore not be tempted by those chocolate biscuits in the back of the cupboard. However, when there is a lack of real nutrients in a meal we ingest we can experience something called 'rebound hunger' and end up having to eat when we probably might not have needed to if we had eaten a proper meal in the first place. We also know that in the state of hunger we tend to make less than ideal choices about what to eat. This is the theory proposed to explain the link between diet soda and weight gain: your body is fooled into 'believing' it has received nutrition and when the subsequent nutrients don't get delivered you are punished with compensatory eating. Ouch! In reality there is unlikely to be a food substitute that comes close to the benefits of eating a diet full of a variety of whole foods.

What about liquid 'foods'?

Take a look at the aisles of large pharmacies for weight-loss products and you'll likely find shelves and shelves of shakes. There are some interesting findings on these little numbers. While it's early days it seems that liquid forms of food provide less satiety than solid foods, which might raise questions over the efficacy of some liquid-based weight-loss programs. It seems even the addition of thickening agents to add bulk to the product and create that sense of fullness may not be effective in actually making the consumer feel they are full. But it's interesting to note the sheer strength of our psychology: just by adding a 'teaspoon' of 'expectation' to the mix our feelings of fullness appear to improve.[9] That is, if the product *claims* it will help you feel full you are more likely to experience increased satiety.

An interesting recent finding is that our expectation of how satiating a food is affects how much we might eat. For example, if we believe that a food is going to fill us up then we are less likely to consume more of it or other foods. The theory is that our taste sensations set up expectations about how filling a food will be, which becomes, in a sense, a self-fulfilling prophecy. You can see how marketing and labelling is going to come into all of this soon![10]

So it seems that even suggestion — just our mere expectation — can affect how much we eat. Tricky stuff! Remember 'conscious eating', so now you are aware of this you have the opportunity to be less influenced by it. More on the power of marketing in Chapter 7.

What about the effect of having eaten?

Sensory-specific satiety (SSS) refers to that feeling of 'hmm, that wasn't as good as I was expecting'. More specifically it's our experience of reduced satisfaction with a meal, from having eaten a food then the follow-on effect of appetite from exposure to more food or flavour. This phenomenon demonstrates the effect of physical stimuli and/or the environment and taste on our eating and hunger.

Here's a great example of how SSS works that many of us can relate to. There's a gorgeous, mouth-watering buffet begging for you to fill your plate to the brim! Let's face it, most of us tend to consume greater amounts of food in this situation; this is largely due to factors such as the variety of food and flavours on offer and potentially how much we have paid. It is this variety that sparks the desire to overeat, in other words the desire to try other foods and tastes overrides our feelings of fullness. We keep going back for more even though we are quite likely already full — that's SSS.

How do we know we are full and how does this signal occur? We have already touched on a few factors but there are many more beyond our mere physiology that can lead to satiety, for example:

- **Meal size. Studies suggest that SSS occurs between two and twenty minutes after exposure to a meal or food. Remember, it takes about twenty minutes for our stomach to empty the food contents into the intestinal canal and for signals of satiety to occur; that is, it takes twenty minutes on average from eating to feel full.**

- **The meal characteristics. For example, sweet and savoury tastes tend to stimulate SSS earlier than other tastes, and more intense-tasting foods also stimulate SSS. Interestingly a variety of tastes appears to increase our food intake, and even the shape of food appears influential. The people you eat with also influence intake (if others finish before us we tend to stop eating) and the order in which you eat your food affects your sense of fullness.**

- **Nutrient composition. As we know, protein stimulates satiety the fastest out of all nutrients, followed by carbohydrates and then fat and alcohol.**

■ Food characteristics, such as the length of time required to chew a food. And those foods often deemed as tasting 'boring' in the early days of a diet — healthy salads, fresh produce — seem to have a strong influence on satiety, which might be why in the first days of moving to a healthy diet many people eat only small amounts.

It's possible that all aspects of food can affect our intake. There is a large amount of research that has been conducted on food intake under various situations, such as how eating with others affects intake, the effect of music while eating, the effect of lighting and so on. You can try to set up an artificial setting to reduce or increase the intake of food depending on what you are seeking to achieve but, at the end of the day, we don't fully understand how all these factors interact with one another in a natural setting. Ultimately, conscious eating is about being aware of what your hand is putting into your mouth. But don't get too bogged down in the minute details.

Ratios of nutrients have a role

It's not merely the presence of a nutrient that can affect us but the ratio of one nutrient to another. For example, the carbohydrate–protein ratios in our diet can affect the production of chemicals in our brain (neurotransmitters, to be precise) called monoamine neurotransmitters. These nifty little numbers are vital for mood stability. It seems that when we experience fluctuations in monoamine levels we can experience depression and other mood disorders. Next we have serotonin, another neurotransmitter involved in mood, which is made from the essential amino acid tryptophan ('essential' referring to the fact that our body can't make this amino acid and instead we must get it via our diet). Now, it's important to not run out and grab a bottle of tryptophan thinking it will cure those down days. The relationship between total protein intake and tryptophan levels in the brain is complex and involves ratios of carbohydrates as well as total protein. It's not so straightforward.

Healthful eating task:
How do taste preferences influence your eating?

This task will help you recognise how our taste preferences can influence not only our current eating patterns but also help plan improvements to our diet.

Task 1: Consider that 80 per cent of salt in our diet comes from processed, refined foods. If a person currently consumes a diet high in refined foods and low in fresh foods and is looking to alter their diet, how might salt impact the transition to a fresh food diet? Write your answer below:

Task 2: Consider the following comment from a person on a diet to reduce body fat. Then list some of the factors that might impact on the success of this person's dietary changes.

> I have been on a weight-loss diet for about four months now. To be honest I really don't enjoy it. The food is bland, I am always hungry and never feel full and I hate eating alone (I can't eat with my husband because it's tempting to eat his meal, it looks a lot more appetising).

4
Learning and its effect on food choice

T his chapter is all about getting to know yourself a bit better. Who doesn't love a little introspection, looking at how both we and others function? One of the most fundamental areas of psychology is learning and this is valuable to any area of human behaviour. Like so much of psychology, learning is based on theories, most of which have held up quite well over the years. Understanding how we have learnt something can be very helpful in determining the best way to unlearn or reshape a behaviour that needs a bit of tweaking, so to speak.

We have spent a good deal of time considering all the factors involved in our eating habits and food choices; now let's get to grips with the processes by which our behaviours in relation to food are formed and how we can reshape them where needed.

As a starting point, let's consider memory. Memory itself has an important influence on our learning, and understanding roughly how it works can help to make sense of learning theories. After all, if you can't hold something in your memory you can't put in place learning processes. Our memory system is a bit like a fishing net, all interconnected; some might say it's also like a mind map (with its interconnecting concepts). As we learn, a new word for example, new neural pathways in our brain are laid down, ideally in relation to other known concepts or events. Figure 5 gives an example of how we might learn that the word 'goldfish' refers to a fish and that it lives in water, that it has gills and that it is generally gold in colour. Of course, each of these concepts has its own string of concepts related to it and our memory of what these mean. And so it goes on. Learning is a bit like a filing system, like a library for example: if we add a book to the library by simply randomly putting it on any shelf it's very unlikely we'll ever see it again, unless by pure luck or accident. Similarly, if we don't associate a concept with anything else — if it floats about on its own without any connections — we won't be able to find it in our memory. Concepts must have associations and other concepts hanging from them, there must be a string or trail to give it some meaning and reference in our memory bank so we can expand on it and recall it when needed.

Figure 5: Mind map of the word 'goldfish'

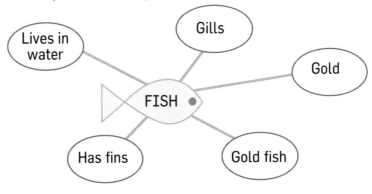

The greatest amount of learning occurs in early childhood, when the brain is still rapidly laying down neural paths, this helps to explain why early eating habits are so important. As we have just discussed, learning and memory are thought to occur best when new concepts are associated to something we already know and understand. Some theories suggest, for example, that children will learn something better if it is directly related to experiences within their own lives. So if we were teaching a child how to subtract we might use toy trucks. The important thing to take from this is that memory (and learning) requires association and systems that are linked.

How learning happens

Theories on learning (or conditioning) are quite complex. The following is a brief outline of the main concepts — classical conditioning, instrumental conditioning and the social learning theory — and how they apply to eating habits. These three theories alone cover much of what is believed about how we learn even though they come from different perspectives.

Classical conditioning

One of the early theories on how we learn was called *classical conditioning*. This form of learning involves associations between events and outcomes. If you have a fear of spiders or a phobia of escalators then classical conditioning might help explain it. The man considered the 'bigwig' of classical conditioning was Ivan Pavlov. Many of us are familiar with his experiment in making a dog salivate to the sound of a bell. In short, Pavlov showed some meat to a dog, which naturally salivated in response to the sight of this morsel, as you would expect. Being a clever soul, Pavlov rang a bell just prior to the meat being presented each time, and guess what? With time the dog salivated to the sound of the bell even before the meat was presented. Furthermore, Pavlov found that the dog would salivate to the sound of the bell even when the meat was not presented.

We see examples of this form of learning every day. Here are a few examples you might relate to.

- **Think back to when you last smelt ground coffee beans and how you then suddenly wanted a coffee.**

- **What do you do when someone holds a balloon to your face that isn't tied up? You squint in preparation for the rush of wind in your eyes.**

- **Do you know of someone who touches wood or paper when they are trying not to jinx themselves?**

- **Does your mouth water when you watch someone cut a lemon, or even just at the thought of it?**

All of these conditions elicit a response from our past experiences and expectations of what might happen.

So you can see that a stimulus paired with another part of the environment causes a reaction or conditioned response. That is classical conditioning.

Classical conditioning can be applied to food preferences. For example, an infant might eat a meal that is too lumpy for them and causes them to gag. If that meal happens to contain broccoli the child might develop a dislike for broccoli. This can also be the case if a meal is eaten in an unpleasant environment — say it is rushed, or people are arguing. An association between dinner and unpleasant activities could develop.

Classical conditioning, however, is a very passive view of learning.

It tends to view humans as largely acting on instinct and nervous system activity. So let's move on to our next theory, which is similar but adds a number of levels by looking at the effect of punishers (sounds nasty but it's not meant to be!) and rewards.

Instrumental conditioning

Instrumental conditioning, also known as operant psychology, grew out of classical conditioning. Harvard psychologist B.J. Skinner found that our behaviour can be altered (increased and decreased) by pleasant or unpleasant events. Instrumental learning involves reinforcement (such as a reward) or 'punishment', not just physical but also withdrawal of something we want or like. According to this theory learning involves an action and an outcome. If we behave well, for example, we might be rewarded. Conversely if we behave badly we could lose a privilege or treat. Children quickly learn relationships between food and their behaviour. Here are a few examples you might relate to.

- **Offering ice-cream when dinner has been eaten.**

- **Removing a favourite toy from a child who has been badly behaved.**

- **Teaching a dog to sit by using treats.**

- **Getting your partner to do a chore by complimenting them on how well they do it.**

- **Allowing children to use electronic games after they have done their homework.**

- **Going to work so that we can be paid.**

The list goes on. Every day we do things because of something we have learnt! In particular, children and students are learning huge amounts of new tasks and knowledge.

UNDERSTANDING THE IMPACT OF REWARDS AND 'PUNISHERS'

Before we move on it's important to say that some of the examples are not necessarily effective strategies. Rewards must be used wisely; all too often they can become the motivator for our behaviour and the actual action becomes of secondary importance. For example, rewarding a child for eating a particular vegetable can reduce their actual enjoyment of the vegetable and increase the desire for the reward. More on this later.

Here are the four possible strategies to amend behaviour.

1. *A reward to increase a behaviour.* Also referred to as positive reinforcement, this is used when you are trying to increase a good behaviour by giving a pleasant reward. Simple: do right and be rewarded.

2. *A positive punisher to decrease a behaviour.* Positive punishment happens when you want a behaviour to decrease by giving a punisher after it occurs. In this case it might be easier to consider the use of the word 'positive' to be positive insofar as it reduces an undesirable behaviour. In other words: do wrong and be punished. So far so good — most of us use these two strategies without thinking.

3. *A negative reinforcer to increase a behaviour.* Negative reinforcement happens when you want a behaviour to increase by removing something unpleasant after the behaviour. If this is a bit tricky for you, try taking 'negative' to mean 'removal'. For example, you want your staff to take on more responsibility so you advise them they will not be in trouble for taking a risk.

4. *A punisher to decrease a behaviour.* Negative punishment occurs when we want a behaviour to decrease as a result of removing something we enjoy after the unwanted behaviour has occurred. Importantly we distinguish negative reinforcement by the desired outcome to *increase* a behaviour and a negative punisher to *decrease* a behaviour.

Mmm, it's all starting to sound a bit like Dr Seuss! But don't worry, you're not being trained to be a psychologist here, so all you really need to grasp is that a reward and a punisher can either increase a wanted behaviour or decrease an unwanted one. If you can really come to grips with this sort of detail you will have unlocked a powerful tool for behaviour modification, but it's not easy and takes years to learn how to apply it effectively.

Broadly, learning highlights the importance of enjoyable meal routines in fostering healthy eating attitudes and habits. After all, if what we learn throughout our lives results in our behaviours, then getting this right as early as possible will mean there's a far greater chance our behaviours will foster lifelong healthy outcomes. It may also influence the acceptance of foods. A positive re-enforcer increases the likelihood that a behaviour will be repeated — but be aware that this can have both positive and negative results. How many of us as parents have fallen into the trap of encouraging our little ones to eat vegetables by promising the reward of ice-cream afterwards? If we are lucky this might lead to some small increase in vegie eating, but it's more likely to increase their love of ice-cream. If we consider ice-cream as a reward for the good behaviour of eating your vegies, the treat can become such a strong motivator that our little cherubs misbehave in order to get the treat. Most of us know children who will hold out eating anything they don't like until the promise of ice-cream afterwards is made, or who throw a tantrum until the ice-cream is forthcoming.

The same applies for those trying to change their eating habits. So many of us believe that we must deprive ourselves, punish ourselves for our errant ways. If we consider the many ways in which we and others do this we can begin to see just how many strategies work against us. Research shows that taste perception plays a role in moving from an unhealthy way of eating (consuming processed foods high in salt, unhealthy fats and unwanted compounds and low in fresh ingredients and variety). In order to create a shift that is more likely to be permanent, strategies that focus on positive outcomes and the use of *appropriate* rewards is integral. The harder but more long-term rewarding alternative is to create a positive environment around meals that can increase the likelihood of acceptance of new foods and new tastes.

Likewise a punisher (which aims to reduce bad behaviour) can be both positive and negative; that is, it can reduce the occurrence of bad behaviour but also inadvertently reduce the occurrence of a desirable behaviour. For example, if we have a preference for sweet foods, reducing our exposure to them can reduce the desirability of the food; alternatively, *not* creating a positive eating environment while eating foods that are new may reduce the enjoyment of the food and lead to rejection of the food later.

There is a great story is of a man who was being bothered by a group of young boys bouncing a ball against his wall of his apartment. He decided to pay each boy a sum for coming each day and bouncing the ball for a period of time. A few days later he offered the boys a much lower sum of money, after which the boys stopped coming. Rewards can be very tricky!

Despite the subtlety of our actions, they have significant outcomes. It is a complex matter and resists simplification, but ultimately food should be enjoyed for its own qualities and its positive social influence in our lives and not be seen as a chore, a science or a reward. It sustains us, it is us and we should approach it in the manner of many southern Europeans: enjoy every bite in a relaxed manner.

Social learning theory

Finally, *social learning theory*, also known as imitation, is an important aspect of learning. While the previous forms of learning centre on relationships between a person and events, imitation is a more vicarious way of learning, involving mere observation. We all learn best from role models we like, are attracted to, who are repeatedly available, are important to us or similar to us. Children tend to model their behaviour on those closest to them, and commonly on those who are the same sex as them. Imitating behaviour appears to start as early as the first week of life. A child's imitation skills rapidly improve to the point where we can't get enough of teaching them to do funny or clever things. Considering how much of our children's behaviour can be modelled, it is so important that we set positive examples for them when it comes to eating habits and attitudes. This is also why there has been much attention on the advertising of junk food towards children.

Learning from others quickly extends beyond the home as young children are exposed to a wider circle of people, many of whom exert strong influences on a child's learning. An interesting study looked at the influence of 'silent teacher modelling'. The teacher modelled eating habits for the children to see — but didn't say anything — and the results of the children's acceptance of new foods was recorded. Findings showed that this form of modelling had only a limited effect with a rapid drop-off over time; in other words, there was only a very short temporary effect. The same study also found that a teacher modelling with enthusiasm ('Mmm! I love mangoes!') could maintain new food acceptance for far longer. One fascinating finding was that if the teacher was competing with a peer model, even enthusiastic teacher-modelling was no longer effective in encouraging new food acceptance.[1] As we all know, peers have a very strong influence over children. Additionally, gender differences were evident, with girls more influenced by the peer model. Such snippets might give us clues to the best way of encouraging children to accept new foods: rather than the use of rewards, perhaps an enthusiastic model might be useful.

Keep in mind that adults are not immune to social learning — if we were then we wouldn't see high-profile athletes and celebrities endorsing a plethora of products, nor would the sales of magazines that adorn their covers with celebs sell so well if we weren't influenced by their lives. We'll look at marketing in a later chapter, but for now, ask yourself how many times you have bought a product or a food simply because an athlete portrays themselves using it? Of course not all of us fall for this, but most do at some point!

Healthful eating task:
Identify different learning methods

The aim of this task is to distinguish between the different methods of learning in relation to food habits, in order to better understand how a habit has come about, which in turn affects how to unlearn behaviours.

Next to each statement overleaf write in which of the forms of learning are likely to have been a factor (there could be more than one).

Table 6: Learning methods

Behaviour	Form of learning
I get Mum to buy a cereal that has my favourite athlete on it because I do a lot of sport.	
I love chocolate; it always makes me feel happier when I am sad.	
I remember getting food poisoning after sushi once and now I can't even bear the smell of raw fish.	
My mother use to make us eat cooked liver, and if we didn't we would have to have it as leftovers the next day. Now I absolutely loathe the stuff.	
We used to have to drink milk at school, but by the time we got to it in summer it was warm and often curdled. I still can't drink cows' milk.	
If I complain enough about being tired my husband will eventually just order pizza. I have him well trained.	
I eat this muesli bar because it has a tick on it that says it's healthy.	
I love salt and vinegar crisps; Mum always had a pack in the cupboard when I was a kid.	
I use low-fat products because the adverts tell you how bad fat is for you.	
I love desserts, always have ever since I was a kid when I was a fussy eater.	

Flavour is learnt

We've looked at how eating habits can be learnt. Let's now delve a little deeper and look at flavour. We have already looked at taste and how that works but there is a little more to flavour. Flavour involves a stimulus such as food or drink that activates several of our senses, each of which differs anatomically in terms of how it functions and activates. The main sense for flavour includes:

- smell (olfaction)
- taste
- chemosensation (chemical reaction, that is, via touch or irritation).

Some foods activate the same receptor but have a different dimension, for example aspartame and sugar have only a different timeline of response; that is, one hits our taste senses more quickly than the other and this allows us to determine the difference.

Our understanding of flavour is something we learn. For example, where you grew up will influence whether you identify benzaldehyde as almond or cherry flavour (those who grew up in the United States will tend to pick it as cherry and those in Australia as almond). We also know that infants prefer tastes their mother consumed while pregnant — it's amazing to think that flavour appears both to cross the placenta and occur in breastmilk.

Flavour-consequence learning

When applying behavioural learning theories such as classical, or Pavlovian, learning to taste preferences and food habits, this is best demonstrated via flavour-consequence learning (FCL). FCL is said to occur when a flavour creates a hedonic response after having been eaten. We begin to get a sense of ways we can alter our experience with food as a method of reshaping our eating habits for health.

If we look at Figure 6 we can see that flavours initially cause a response such as liking, but when flavours are *repeatedly* associated with a food or drink this can lead to higher-level responses such as satiation. You can see that this might be important in encouraging us to adjust our taste preferences by repeated pairing of liked and new foods both to improve the enjoyment of and increase compliance with the new food options. Remember, we are trying to override old behaviours with new, reshaped ones. You can see that simply ceasing to eat all foods you love but feel you shouldn't eat might not be the best route for success. In fact, doing this can for some simply be the beginning of failure. After all, how long can you keep it up if you really don't enjoy your new diet? Some refer to this as inhibition eating, where we try to inhibit the desire to eat a certain food. Research tends to suggest that as a form of restriction it is not effective over the long term. Something we'll look at later is emotions and eating but it's worth noting now that stress itself can increase both food intake and body weight just in relation to the hormones we secrete when stressed. As we will see, food restriction in itself can be a stressor.

The post-ingestive effects of food

The effect that a food has on us after we have eaten it is obviously an important factor in whether we enjoy and seek out that food in the future. There are a number of documented post-ingestive effects of food; for example, there is a positive relationship between liking and the energy density of food. That is, we tend to like more energy-dense foods (yes, those fatty foods). This strengthens the theory of hedonic pleasure being a factor in the love of fatty foods many of us experience. This also makes sense of why so many of us enjoy coffee despite its

Figure 6: Classical learning and flavour-consequence learning in action[2]

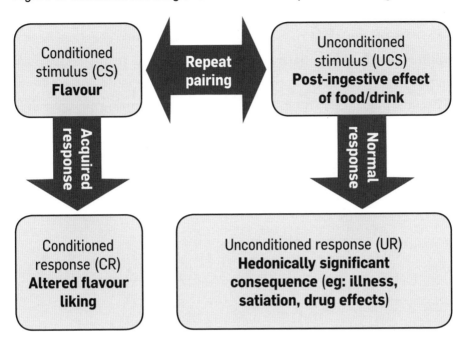

bitter taste — it is the post-ingestive effect on our physiology of the pharmacological compounds such as caffeine that creates a positive experience, overriding the initial taste response.

This area of food preferences is still being studied and data is quite sparse at this point, but you are sure to see more research hitting the press in the near future.

Other factors in learning

In food psychology, *exposure* is regarded as a form of learning. Repeated, unreinforced taste exposure to a food is believed to increase our preference for that food. To date studies on this are limited, though you may have seen this employed as a way to overcome food issues in children or even in adults who have food neophobia (fear of new foods). There have been numerous TV programs about children and their 'bad eating behaviours' where the behaviour expert simply repeatedly exposes the child to a new food to get them to eventually eat it without a fight. They make it look so easy, but the reality is that such initiatives are often best implemented by people the child doesn't know. The same might apply for us big people who are adjusting our unhealthy eating habits; working with an independent person can make the transition more successful. After all, most of us know what we should be doing but it's the doing that is hardest.

5
Changing behaviours

We've focused a lot on the importance of reshaping behaviour. Now let's look at how we can achieve this by first considering habits. What are they, how do they come about and, the biggie, how do we change the ones that don't serve us well? The area of behavioural change is potentially going to be one of the central factors in the success of our eating goals.

Do old habits really die hard?

We form habits when behaviours we have learnt become so ingrained we barely need to think about them. Some examples might include:

- opening the fridge every time you are bored
- adding salt to your meal before tasting it
- going to the gym on a certain day each week
- putting on pants starting with the same leg each time
- biting your nails when you are stressed

101

- **piling up your plate at the buffet**
- **eating the kids' leftovers**
- **buying fast food when you are at the mall**
- **choosing a cake over fruit**
- **buying one brand because you know it**
- **eating chocolate when you feel tired**
- **drinking alcohol with your meal.**

And so on. There are many habits and they vary from one person to the next.

Some of our habits can become less than helpful. Many athletes develop routines and behaviours that might border on superstitious. Believing that you have to be first back on the tennis court after a break, for example, or touching a lucky charm, having to wear a certain number or piece of clothing, and so on. There can be a fine line between a habit or behaviour being helpful or affecting us adversely by negatively impacting on our lives. A habit that affects our daily living by, for example, preventing us from going about our usual activities is likely to be a problem.

How are habits formed?

Hands up those of you who have tried a new diet. At first you feel really psyched and motivated — that first phase of habit formation is the honeymoon stage. But as the days go on you start to hit the wall and your enthusiasm ebbs away. This second stage is pivotal. Writing in *Forbes* magazine, mental training expert Jason Selk looked at habit formation and suggested that in order to build a stronger base of habit formation we must 'fight through' by recognising we have hit the reality stage.[1] We need to ask ourselves how we will feel if we stick with the changes and how we will feel if we give up. And failing this, we should create a vision of our actual life if we give up now, seeing ourselves in that life and trying hard to feel what that would be like.

Fiona Cosgrove from Wellness Coaching Australia suggests that we need to consider:

- **the benefit of staying the same versus the reasons for changing**
- **the issues about staying the same versus the concerns about changing.**[2]

If we consider both these issues we can go forward more consciously to reach our goals.

There are many things that can get in the way of change. Barriers to change can be:

- **BEHAVIOURAL, that is things that we do or can't do**
- **SITUATIONAL, such as our jobs or families**
- **COGNITIVE, being thoughts that can work against us**
- **EMOTIONAL, including our fears.**

Selk suggests that there are three main obstacles to habit formation.

- **DISCOURAGEMENT in the form of overthinking results that aren't what you expected, listening to negative self-talk or negative talk from others.**
- **DISRUPTION from life events that can be as minor as a public holiday through to illness.**
- **THE SEDUCTION OF SUCCESS as Selk puts it; that is, overestimating the process of what led to your changes.**

Still, assuming you stay on track you will eventually hit the mark and the new behaviour in itself will become a habit. But while the process of habit formation can have a quick and easy feel to it, we all know that's not the case. Old habits can take a great deal of time to change, or even hang about and possibly compete while new ones are being formed. Selk suggests that 'greatness requires sacrifice ... good habits require constant commitment'. Theories on habit formation suggest that they are so difficult to remove because they are entrenched in our neural circuits. You could question whether they ever really leave you or if they are simply overwritten if time allows.

> **Tip:** Be kind to yourself. The process of change doesn't generally happen overnight (unless you experience an extreme life event). It can be a process of two steps forward, one back, but as long as the general direction is forward that is what counts.

How to change your habits

If you check out what researchers have to say, there are a number of strategies that appear to be important in new habit formation. Repetition of the new behaviour (and as we will see there is a critical time period) is important. If habits are indeed ingrained in our neural circuitry then writing over them as often as we can is likely to be a rewarding strategy. In essence, we need to practise the new behaviour at every opportunity! For example, if you are trying to reduce your portion size you would ideally do this everywhere you eat: at home, at family and friends' homes, when eating out, and so on. Spreading the new behaviour like this will reinforce the new habit. Excluding situations can slow the process and act as a distraction.

Next, having a strong set of strategies is important and this should include, as one of the most influential, self-monitoring. You then need a selection of the following (depending on the individual and the situation).

- **Formation of strong goals.**
- **Regular feedback you can give yourself and from others who might be involved on how you are going.**
- **Re-evaluations of your goals.**

In other words, you need to be clear on where you are heading, how you intend to get there and how you will know if you are on the right track. Self-monitoring appears to be a very strong factor in the success of change. You might need to create a program or have a program created for you; either way it needs to address each of these factors.

Health coaches commonly use rating scales, working with their clients to self-rate on a scale of one to ten. Health and wellness coaches will also encourage people to create short-term (weekly) goals and medium-term goals (three-monthly) as well as an overall vision.

'Vision' is a word that gets bandied about a lot in motivational circles. However, having a vision of who or what you want to be does not mean you simply have a one liner (for example, 'I am going to be healthier'). Wellness coaches such as Fiona Cosgrove suggest that having a vision involves asking yourself:

- Who is the ideal me?

- How far away am I from my ideal self? Rate this on a scale of one to ten and then reassess with this scale once you are closer to your goal.

- What does the ideal me look and feel like? Describe this person, what he or she does, the values they hold, the activities they do, the attitudes they exhibit.

- Why is being this person important to me?

Once you have answered these you will begin to reveal some of those values we looked at in Chapter 2. Of course, these will likely be broader personal values and if your goal is to be healthier they will be centered around these — values around healthy eating, being active, having time to relax, being happy and so on. On p. 108 you'll have a chance to create and write down your own personal vision in the next Healthful Eating Task.

SMART goals

Once you have a clear vision, the next step is defining your goals. A well-known approach to goal formation is the SMART model, which states that goals should be specific, measureable, appealing, realistic and within a set timeframe. Let's go through each of these now.

- Based on the vision you will detail for yourself on p. 108, your goals should be specific and descriptive, for example, 'I am going to cut down my serving sizes over a month so that I am not overeating to the point where I am overfull.' Being too vague can be a recipe for failure.

- Goals should be measurable so that you can assess how you are going. Using the above example we could measure our level of fullness by a self-rating scale (see the self-monitoring table in the Healthful Eating Task box on p. 109).

- Our goals should appeal to us. It's far more motivating to work towards something we want rather than something we believe we should be doing or that someone else thinks should be our goal.

- At the same time goals need to be realistic. Setting lofty goals can be a signal that we aren't committed to our change or fear it in some way. For example, 'I am going to lose 10 kilograms (22lb) in a month' is unrealistic (the body tends to give up around half a kilo (1lb) a week) and can quickly set us up for failure.

- Last, goals should have a timeframe so you can assess how well you are going and if your goal needs tweaking. Even goals can need to be changed.

When creating your goals consider the obstacles that might be in your way (revisit 'How are habits formed?' on p. 102 if you need to). Review what attributes and abilities you have that will help or hinder. Think about what will keep you motivated and what will be your distractions. And focus on creating strategies that meet/address these so that you can increase your chances of success.

Undertake the following Healthful Eating Task to put all this together.

Healthful eating task:
Set your vision and goals

Write your answer for each of the following questions. Take time to consider your answer and ensure it is in line with your own goals and vision — not anyone else's. You might wish to photocopy this page and place it on your fridge or other prominent place so you can refer to it whenever you need to.

Q: What is the health-related goal you want to achieve from healthy eating?

Q: What will you look and feel like when you achieve this? Describe the vision of yourself when you achieve your goals.

Q: What areas of your life will you need to make amendments to in order to achieve your goals and vision?

Self-monitoring

Use the following table to monitor yourself over the next three weeks as you progress towards your goal. Remember, use a scale of 1 to 10, with 10 being 'I've reached my goal!'.

	Starting Point	End Week 1	End Week 2	End Week 3
How close are you to your goal?				
How close do you feel to the goal, i.e. how close is your vision to becoming a reality?				
How much effort have you put into making changes?				
How important is this change to you?				
How confident are you that you can achieve this goal?				

Medium-term goals

As we discussed earlier, medium-term goals are goals that cover the next three months. In the space below, list three medium-term goals that will assist you in moving towards your vision. Alongside each goal, list a strategy you will use to achieve that goal. Then place an asterisk next to the one goal you feel is the most important — this is the goal you will work on for the first month; then move on to the second medium-term goal in the following month, while still keeping the first in motion.

Consider any requirements and strengths you will need to be mindful of as you strive for change. Also think about any barriers to change you might encounter.

The critical stage of change

A study of 1289 people conducted by the Australian Psychological Society found that 98 per cent of the participants who had attempted to change their diet reported 'some success', while 22 per cent reported that their change lasted less than a few weeks or months. A further 26 per cent of subjects were able to maintain their changed behaviour for more than six months. However, only 12 per cent who had amended their eating habits less than six months ago were still maintaining the new behaviour.[3]

The study concluded that the 'four to six month stage in change appears to be a critical time for strengthening a commitment to the new behaviour'.[4] Other studies support that if a behaviour is maintained for up to six months it is more likely to continue.

Tips to improve success

Sticking to your guns will be a challenge at some point, so it's important to remember that compliance is generally best where we have reasonably clear and achievable guidelines. One of the truly great authorities on food psychology, Brian Wansink, has shown that while weight-loss coaches can really kick start you in the right direction, long-term compliance (beyond two months) seems to wane. What's even more interesting is that when people are given a long list of tips to use to improve their eating they stick less to this than if they are instructed to only select a handful. Even if people are given the option to choose just a few strategies of their own, almost all would rather choose from a list provided. You'd have to say that we are better at doing just a few things that we know will work than trying to do it all.[5]

Wansink has an excellent website with lots of tips about how to become a better eater (see 'Resources', p. 195). In essence he suggests you need to do the following:

- Focus on just one goal at a time.

- Choose three changes that will work for you.

- Create a simple 30-day initial plan that works for you.

- Ensure you stick to your plan.

- But modify the plan if you need to and go on to the next 30 days.

A simple plan

We have looked at using a vision plan, now take your page with your vision and goal and, using a calendar write at the top of each month the goal you are going to focus on that month. Then for each day write in an example where you have achieved this or a note about why you haven't.

Review each month before you create your plan for the next month by reviewing your vision plan. You may need to adjust it or redesign and replace it, but keep the old copies. Write notes to yourself about how you went, what worked well and why, and what didn't and what you will do about it on your vision plan. You might find there are some months you need to repeat your goal as you don't feel it has become enough of a habit.

Altering your eating habits

Below is a list of tips and strategies you can use in altering your eating habits to reach the goal you have written down. Select just a couple that 'hit home' for you and write them on your vision sheet or calendar to remind you that this is your plan.

Portion size changes

- Use smaller plates and bowls.
- Use smaller serving utensils.
- Have a glass of water before you eat.
- Do your assessment of hunger and fullness.
- Leave a small amount of food on your plate so no one refills your plate.
- Drink from tall, narrow glasses and cups, as they appear bigger.
- Consider how much you will eat before you begin rather than eating as you go.
- Start eating last so that you eat less socially.
- Don't let the waiting staff clear your table so you can see how many servings you have consumed.
- Sit at a table away from the buffet so you aren't continually exposed to huge amounts of varied dishes.
- When you do go to a buffet select just two dishes first and avoid mounds of food — low and flat servings are best.
- Watch packaging and don't assume that a packet, tin, jar, etc, is a serving — you might need to use much less.

- Move less healthy food options to the back of the fridge or cupboard and make them super hard to access or even better don't have them in the house.

- In the same vein bring the healthy foods such as fruit, etc, to the front and make them easy to access.

- Separate leftovers into small containers to avoid being tempted to eat everything in one go.

- Where possible, dish up meals rather than eating buffet style.

- Put food onto a plate or bowl, this particularly includes premade foods.

- Eat fruit before you snack.

- Serve up your meals with a salad and eat that first.

- While you prepare dinner nibble on a carrot or a handful of nuts, or something healthy yet filling.

Eating habits

- Tell others about your new healthier eating habits and enlist their positive support.

- Select the top eating habit you think gets in the way of healthy eating and start from there.

- Use a shopping list when grocery shopping.

- Avoid making food choices when hungry (avoid getting hungry).

- Find a menu-planning app.

- Create a menu of each week's meals for the next month.

- Plan meals the night before to avoid making rash decisions.

- Ask yourself if you really need that unhealthy option or if you are eating mindlessly.

- Stop picking at others' meals such as the kids'.

Putting it into action

As we saw in the previous chapter, the way in which we learn things can have a strong influence over how easy it is to unlearn or change that learnt behaviour. In order to affect a change we need to understand how a behaviour has come about. Let's see if we can piece together a holistic approach with which to change eating habits.

We need to consider five factors.

1. First, the way in which we have gained our food preferences, that is, were they learnt or are they innate?

2. Secondly, how long has the behaviour been with us?

3. How often is it reinforced?

4. What is the end goal?

5. And last but not least, what is your plan of attack for getting to your end goal? This will address the answers to points 1 to 4.

Each of these will be influential in affecting positive changes.

Here's an example. I have decided I want to stop drinking so much coffee.

1. How have I learnt my preference for coffee? I think I have learnt this through social reinforcement, when I am out or with friends I drink coffee and now I drink it all the time.

2. How long have I been drinking coffee? I started when I was seventeen and I am now 34, so seventeen years. That's a long time; hmm, might not be a simple transition.

3. How often do I drink coffee and really enjoy it? Hmm, well I absolutely love my morning coffee and I think it helps me to get going. I drink the rest through the day, and

I think this is more out of habit. I wonder if the caffeine will also be a factor in making my change?

4. My end goal? To get down to three cups a day.

5. My plan of attack is to have a full-strength coffee first thing in the morning for a month. In the second month I am going to just have one coffee a day at home and from there slowly reduce my coffees outside of home and possibly swap to decaffeinated as I know when I meet my friends I won't be able to resist a coffee no matter how many I have had that day. Eventually I would like to swap a coffee for a fresh juice or a smoothie and/or herbal tea.

Healthful eating task:
Behavioural adjustments

Select three strategies from the lists on pp. 113–114 and apply them for a week. Then select another three for week two and another three for week three. Write them in the chart below.

	Week 1	Week 2	Week 3	**Your notes:** record how consistent you were each week
Strategy 1				
Strategy 2				
Strategy 3				

Habits hardest to change

Before we move on let's spend some time considering which of our habits/behaviours are our most stubborn. Some habits die harder than others. Table 7 outlines how resistant behaviours are to change according to how they were learnt. As you can see, the hardest of all to alter are those we learn unconsciously, as in the case of innate preferences for sweet tastes, followed by those learnt via early learning experiences.

Table 7: Resistance levels according to mode of learning[6]

Different forms of learning involved in food habit formation and the extent to which the resulting habits are resistant (+) to change or not (-).

Mode of learning	Resistance to change
Imprinting and condition (pre- and peri-natal)*	+++
Praise, reward and punishment (early childhood; parents or others)	++
Imitation (childhood and puberty; parents, peers, idols)	$\pm$
'Sensory' learning (lifelong; complexity, boredom, exposure)*	++
Cognitive learning (adulthood; advice, labelling, risk perception)	- , +

$\pm$ = more or less

- , + = in some cases, not in others

* = innate, largely implicit and unconscious habit formation

Take, for example, our salty taste perception and liking, which is believed to be largely a factor of learnt experiences.[7] Strategies to change this need to be formulated based on this process. Potentially, the effectiveness of the strategy depends on its relationship to the method of initial learning. As we can see from Table 7, sensory learning is somewhat resistant to change though less resistant than conditioned learning. Hence it is far easier to alter a preference for salty foods than it is to alter a preference for sweet foods (the latter being innate). And that's perhaps why we find it so hard to give up those sweet treats.

However, these can be overridden more easily during 'sensitive periods' in life, such as early childhood, late adolescence coinciding with independent living, major changes such as divorce or spousal death, or pregnancy. So never say never ...

Studies also suggest in the case of where we have learnt an eating behaviour from watching others, or cognitive learning (education), that 'unlearning' may be best done in the same way as the initial learning. For example, habits gained by imitation (copying) or cognitive learning (for example, education) may be best changed by reasoning and cognitive information or by the example of significant role models.

Eating and habits

Studies suggest that habit is one of the most influential aspects of our eating behaviour. It also seems that our habitual behaviour is quite different from non-habitual behaviour in that it requires little information for a decision, our intentions aren't helpful in determining what we will do in the end, and habitual behaviour is strongly influenced by situational cues (the factors around us at the time). The capacity for us to self-regulate dieting is one of the many behaviours that appears to dilute over time.

Again, the area of habit changing in food psychology is fairly new and there really isn't enough research out there to give you any conclusive evidence or strategies other than the few mentioned here. Suffice to say, it's important to understand which of your behaviours escapes your attention, how they came about and what factors influence them; then consider how you are going to go forward from there.

Studies recommend the following:

1. Determine your unwanted eating habits.
2. List the factors that spark them off.
3. Change the situation and environment around you, in particular the things that trigger your unwanted habitual eating habits.
4. Consciously work towards being conscious of your amended behaviour, and be mindful of what you are eating and why (at least until the new habit is secure). This might mean keeping track by charts or reviewing how you are going at certain points or reporting to a professional.

We have already looked at much of this, so let's now turn our attention to the cues that spark the habit or your triggers. This is an important aspect that we haven't as yet covered. Smokers will be very familiar with this idea — when trying to give up smoking most will say that being out socially is a huge trigger for the desire to smoke. Eating habits can also be sparked off by triggers, some of which we have considered such as the mere presence of food, the social occasion, the environment and so on. But you can be more specific. Try to make a list of some of the triggers that lead you to making bad food choices. They may range from:

- having an argument with a certain person
- a certain level or type of stress
- a time of the day
- a place in your home
- a TV show
- TV adverts
- an activity.

Make a list of your triggers and then write out some strategies to defuse them. You may, for example, find that sitting down to watch a cooking show straight after dinner makes you hanker for dessert. Try not watching this show at that time and record it instead. You can use this as one of your strategies in your vision plan.

Controlling ourselves

We will now spend a bit of time focusing on the area of control in relation to our eating. You often hear people refer to others who struggle with healthy eating habits as 'lacking willpower' or 'having no self-control' and so on. But the reality is it's just not that simple. Having already considered the myriad influences on our food choices, preferences and intake you will have some understanding of this, but our ability to inhibit our desire to eat is in a league of its own, as we will see.

Let's start with a demonstration of how strong our habits can be, in particular habits that are so entrenched we are barely aware of them. This will show you that our behaviour is less under our control than some of us may think.

Understanding automatic behaviour

Behaviours that are said to be automatic happen without us being fully aware of them. They start without warning and we often have little control over them. Automatic behaviours are very efficient, they demand very little of our attention or effort — they can be sneaky things. Remember the classic driving example we mentioned earlier? You drive part of the way somewhere then realise you've been on autopilot for most of the trip. That's what an automatic behaviour feels like.

So what about eating? Logically we can argue that many behaviours needed for survival are automatic or intuitive. We can make the leap, then, that eating (inherent to survival) when food is within our reach is an automatic behaviour. Yes, that's probably obvious, but you might not fully realise just how strong automatic behaviours are, or how unconscious and almost beyond our control they can be.

The strength of automatic behaviour

Here's a simple but fun example of how automatic behaviours occur and how strong their effect is. The Stroop Effect is a great example of how some behaviours can be so automatic that we are not in control of them, and even when we are trying to be conscious of them they still overpower us.

Try this:

1. Look at the grid opposite. Read the words and ignore the colour they are printed in (this exercise is traditionally printed in full colour; we have had to opt for tones given this book is printed in black and white). Time yourself and see how fast you are or simply note how many mistakes you make.

2. Now repeat the task, but this time ignore the written word and name the colour the word is written in, for example 'white', 'grey' or 'black'. Again, time yourself or note the number of errors.

Figure 7: The Stroop Effect

GREY	**BLACK**	WHITE	**WHITE**	BLACK
GREY	BLACK	**GREY**	BLACK	**WHITE**
BLACK	**GREY**	BLACK	BLACK	GREY
WHITE	WHITE	GREY	WHITE	**GREY**
GREY	BLACK	**WHITE**	**WHITE**	BLACK

You should have found that not only do you make more mistakes, but it also takes you longer to attend to the colour as you are trying to *not* read the words. You might be using a script to control your automatic behaviour of reading, for example 'focus on the colour', 'stop reading the word' etc. All of this takes up valuable processing time, and you will likely find that even with practice you will rarely get to the same speed as when simply reading the word. The effort that you have to put in to controlling your urge to read the words can be substantial and you might even feel a sense of stress or notice you have really had to put in some effort.

Reading is so automatic that we can do it without conscious thought or effort and we tend to automatically read words. Automatic behaviours tend to have a combination of the following. They:

- **occur without our knowing (awareness)**
- **start without our efforts**
- **tend to continue once they have started**
- **are efficient and require little attention or effort**

- can be difficult to override

- can be exhausting and taxing.

The Stroop Effect demonstrates this very clearly. We need to be conscious eaters and not eat automatically so we can reach a healthful way of eating and a more mindful way of enjoyable eating. If we can do this we begin to take back control over our health.

Eating as an automatic behaviour

Research seems to support the theory that eating is automatic. For example we know that factors such as the portion size on our plate, what food looks like, how easy food is to access all affect how much and what we eat. However, so often we don't know how much we are eating and we are generally completely unaware of all the factors influencing our eating. Indeed, some nutrition researchers go so far as to suggest that the manner in which our food is presented to us, the marketing, easy access and sheer volume of food on offer is a less than helpful modern-day eating environment; you may have heard the term 'obeseogenic' which reflects this sentiment.

The question then arises: how much control do we have over our eating? It's somewhat scary raising this point, as it might be tempting to use automatic eating patterns as an excuse. But if we consider the Stroop Effect, most of us can improve on our times with practice, even if automatic eating patterns are still evident. Potentially the plateauing of obesity figures in some developed countries also shows us we really can change if we work at it. Ultimately we will still have some control — and remember, we are trying to be 'conscious eaters', part of which is first knowing the effects on our eating and then working with them to create change. That's probably unconsciously why you are reading this book — you want to take more control over your eating habits and lifestyle!

How we make choices

We are all familiar with the image of a devil on one shoulder and an angel on the other, each whispering into the person's ear. But just how do we make a decision and how does this affect what we eat and why?

There are thought to be two main types of decision-making styles: intuitive and reasoned. Having an understanding of the characteristics of both will help you grasp the difference:

An intuitive decision-making style is the style we most commonly use. Its characteristics are that it is:

- fast
- multitasked
- automatic
- effortless
- internal
- often emotional.

In contrast, a reasoned decision-making style is characterised by the following qualities. It is:

- slower
- orderly
- governed by logical rules
- deliberate and conscious
- time involved
- monitored
- often flexible.

At present it's believed that eating and drinking is governed predominantly by intuitive thinking and less by rational processes. In itself this can explain why making changes can be so taxing, slow and challenging. Intuitive decisions are going to be harder to adjust given their speed and how automatic they are to us.

The effect of repetition of food and variety

Most of us know that variety is one of the top recommendations for a healthy diet. However, variety itself appears to have an effect on our intake of food and the choices we make.

A number of studies have shown that variety has the effect of increasing food consumption. The variety of foods on offer at a meal, and also across meals, influences how much we are likely to eat. Offering the same old thing tends to reduce both the amount we eat and how much we enjoy the meal. Of course there are some who can seemingly eat the same thing almost every day with the same degree of enjoyment; in this case, studies tend to suggest that it's the choice that matters. That is, if the person selects that food because they can and not because they have to, then the enjoyment is enhanced. But most of us find monotony a real killer of appetite.

Controlling the urge to eat (and eat ...)

This is something worth understanding. Our ability to inhibit the desire to eat when we shouldn't, or to inhibit eating more than is necessary, is important in the maintenance of a healthy body weight.

It seems those of us who find we barely notice we are overeating accessible, inexpensive, palatable food regularly are likely to gain weight because each of these variables encourages the intake of energy. So far studies suggest that in these situations the sheer pleasure and enjoyment from a meal overrides our desire to control our weight. We could be forgiven for feeling like the cards are stacked against us, but what we need to be aware of is that restriction isn't necessarily the best route to success. Creating negative experiences around eating is never ideal. Reflect on your vision and goal setting and recall that a positive stance is going to be more motivating than if you approach something from a negative perspective. Also, come back to your body cues and use these to reframe your eating style so that you are focused on food and health over food and guilt.

Tip: Stating changes of eating habits in a more positive fashion seems to yield far better outcomes. Your goal, vision and reasons for doing something should be in reference to a positive. Changing your eating so you can lose a few kilos isn't really the best ideal to focus on. Instead, focusing on changing your eating habits so you improve your health, reawaken your body cue awareness and increase vitality is a better ideal and the weight loss is framed within this.

Focus also on your efforts to eat healthy options rather than focusing on restraining yourself from eating, which tends to act as a punishment. Food should be enjoyed and pleasurable, not shrouded in negative emotions.

If you know someone who seems to have been on some form of diet all their adult lives, or someone who is vigilant about what they eat and always seems to be restricting themselves at regular times then you know a 'restrained eater'. It's a term used commonly in nutrition in reference to chronic dieters, people who work hard to control or restrict their food intake, and do so in a cycle of control then relapse.

As in life generally, there can seem to be many factors working against us. Restraining our eating can be one of these. Our impulses to eat food we believe we shouldn't and the amount of cognitive effort (thought) exercised in trying to control these impulses can actually increase our chances of overeating. So when we diet regularly and are confronted with yummy food we really, really want and enjoy, particularly while we are under some cognitive stress (such as trying to restrain ourselves), the result is we are more likely to give into our impulses or wants, not to mention then feeling a whole lot of guilt. Dieting in reality works against us in most cases. 'Why have we been urged to do it for so long?' you ask! Good question — potentially it's got something to do with so many people making so much money from the weight-loss industry.

If you are a restrained eater it's possible that you associate food more commonly with hedonic experiences than those who are not restrained eaters. Put simply, you *really* enjoy food, and it's more than just about fuel for you. Quite possibly you might refer to yourself as 'being addicted to cooking shows', much to the joy of the TV ratings people as you are exactly their target audience. A restrained eater is a person who is also more likely to downgrade or compromise their dieting goal when faced with palatable foods; that is, you might be tempted to make excuses or create trade-offs. So a restrained eater might weigh up their enjoyment of a certain food against the temporary 'breaking' of their diet and consider it worth it for now, vowing to make up for it later.

On the other hand, successful restrained eaters will activate their dieting goal when confronted with temptations. If you are a successful restrained eater you will tend to be better able to relate your health goals to your actual choices and behaviours, aligning them in a way that will increase the likelihood of success. We can see here that this is more in tune with a non-diet approach and is somewhat more of a focus on health.

So, restrained eaters who overall can maintain their healthy body weight tend to also experience less wanting for calorie-dense foods, especially in those moments when they are confronted with such foods. Restrained eaters who haven't experienced overall success and tend to be overweight, by and large, are unable to resist such temptations. In other words, food for some is a trigger that starts positive strategies to making healthy choices and for others it triggers emotional states that may not serve them well and causes an increase in their desire for food.

Tip: Have a think about your eating habits and cues, and try to recognise whether you are a restrained eater — and if so, try to pinpoint which type you are. Now keep the following points in mind:

1. Try not to be too hard on yourself.

2. **Put temptation out of sight to avoid having to restrain yourself.**

3. **Choose simple strategies that don't take too much effort to stick to.**

4. **Eat slowly.**

5. **Choose just one thing to work on first (for example, snacking at night; eating while cooking) and wait till the new habit is well entrenched before you move onto the next target. Remember, your current eating habits didn't happen in a day and aren't likely to change overnight, so don't set yourself up for stress, failure or guilt.**

There's more to it

Ever noticed how exhausting it can be to stick to your eating program at every meal? If you have felt drained by the effort of restraining yourself from foods you would rather eat, you were on the money. The amount of effort required to restrain ourselves from eating when food is present is quite significant. And it appears the effort required to sustain this inhibition is more than most of us can cope with. A great study by Baumeister and colleagues demonstrated just how significant the impact is. The researchers conducted a study on three groups of people:

- Group one could consume freshly baked chocolate chip cookies as they wished.

- Group two were required to resist the cookies and instead were allowed to eat radishes.

- Group three were offered no food at all to consume or refuse.

After the session each participant was required to undergo a mental task in order to determine the degree of fatigue that might have occurred from the food session. Group two — those who were asked to resist — gave up on the mental task considerably earlier than the other two groups. The results suggest that the effort to refuse food takes mental stamina, sufficient to deplete our ability to perform higher cognitive tasks.[8]

Studies also suggest that the more effort required to access a food the less we consume of it. For example, if you had to go downstairs and get a stool from the garden shed, then bring it back into the house just to reach a tiny treat you may well not bother. The context within which our food is provided has important implications for our overall consumption. In Chapter 2 we discussed the placement of products in supermarkets to entice you to buy them.

Tip: When in the supermarket, make sure you check the higher and lower shelves and compare products and prices before you make your selections for purchase.

Sustained effort to consciously control automatic behaviours is limited. It seems we simply can't sustain the effort. We tire and hence our effectiveness reduces in controlling the behaviour. It might also be possible that failure to sustain a diet is not simply a consequence of a lack of willpower but rather a lack of recognition of the strength of automatic behaviours, even in eating, and the effect that fast, accessible food has on our eating habits and cognitive functioning. On the positive side, the effect of effort on eating may be useful for those who need to amend their food intake, for example, by increasing the difficulty of access to food to reduce total food intake.

The way forward

Clearly, being overweight has health implications. However, the assumption that dieting is the answer is questionable. Ask any perpetual dieter if they have found a diet that has worked permanently, and that they have found easy, and there will be few who answer yes. It also seems that conventional weight management has been ineffective given the unintended negative outcomes of the focus on weight, on body satisfaction and so on. And as we have seen, long-term restriction and elimination do not work. In reality, when anyone tells you to eliminate a food group from your diet it is very likely not great advice. We are designed to eat diets that are full of variety and it's our one sure way of getting nutrient diversity and sufficiency.

So what's the answer?

Increasingly, healthcare professionals are working to focus on health rather than illness. In fact, in the United States in recognition of this shift, new weight management systems are emerging based on a more non-diet perspective. We are already familiar with one of these, the Health at Every Size (HAES) program created by Linda Bacon. The HAES website makes for interesting reading, starting with its statement that 'Health at Every Size is the new peace movement'. Those who sign up to the website are asked to take the HAES pledge, which is based on acceptance and respect for varying body sizes and shapes;

flexibility in eating, with an approach that takes into account pleasure, hunger cues and satiety; and rediscovering joy in the movement of your body.

Generally speaking we can't change our gender (generally), age, body type, race or genetics — but we *do* have control over the food we eat, the fluid we drink, the amount of activity we undertake and our habits.

6
Eating, emotions, personality and motivation

There is pretty clear evidence that an increasing number of nutrients and compounds in our food can influence our mood. One of the best examples of a food that can affect our mood would have to be … yes, you guessed it, chocolate. There are compounds in chocolate, such as theobromine and caffeine, that influence our mood and behaviour. Studies show that milk chocolate can reduce the level of anxiety for a person who suffers from high levels of anxiety, while cheese and crackers appear to provide an energised feeling for those who have lowered levels of anxiety.[1]

We also know that in some situations we will overeat when we experience negative feelings, more so if there is food we want to eat at the ready. One study also suggested that some of us may eat more when we are angry. Clearly, eating, mood and emotions are closely intertwined for many of us. This is the focus of this chapter.

The effect of stress on eating

We have looked at neural circuits in previous chapters and talked about reprogramming but let's spend some time looking at the nervous system (NS). The NS is the control centre or the central processing unit of the body. The nervous system can be broken down into many parts; however, our concern is with what's called the parasympathetic nervous system. The parasympathetic NS is responsible for our response to threats and fear, commonly referred to as the 'fight or flight' response, which influences many body systems including the heart, eyes, bladder and gastro-intestinal system (GIT). In times of stress our parasympathetic NS will turn off the stomach to direct much needed energy to muscle, dilate the pupils so we can better see the threat, speed up the heart rate so we have blood pumping to muscle, and switch off the bladder. Ta-daa, we are ready to fight or run for the hills.

We'll come back to this concept of how our stress response affects eating. For now, just remember that the standard response to stress includes our GIT slowing and we eat less.

Emotional influences on food choice

The influence of food over our emotions is an area of ongoing interest. You hear some people say they are 'an emotional eater' — for some this means eating more when they are upset while others eat less when stressed. Before we go further, let's quickly look at a few terms commonly used in relation to our emotions, just so we know exactly what we are referring to.

- **MOOD** is a psychological state we experience that lasts at least several minutes, often longer, and involves energy, tension and pleasure; as opposed to
- **EMOTIONS**, which are said to be less specific, less intense and tend to be triggered less by specific events or stimuli.

It's clear that a number of nutrients can affect our mood, as we saw with chocolate. However, does our mood affect our food choices? Much of the research in this area is focused on our ability to inhibit or restrain ourselves from consuming unhealthy food, plus decision-making strategies and how they influence food choices. The actual emotional side tends to receive a little less focus.

A good example of food affecting mood and emotions is the change that occurs from before to *after* eating a meal. When we are in a state of hunger we can be aroused to find food, and at these times we often feel irritable. Children are excellent examples of this: just delaying a meal by ten minutes can result in a cranky child. Children have a limited supply of stored body energy and can reliably become cranky after three or more hours of non-eating. Studies have shown that our emotions towards food are quite stable and less open to change (at least by those around us). However, there is enormous variation in the impact of food from one person to the next.

Emotional eating

Are you an emotional eater? There are two psychological tests to help you answer this question, the Dutch Eating Behaviour Questionnaire and the Intuitive Eating Scale. Both questionnaires are included in the appendices (see p. 183). Such questionnaires rate you on scales regarding your eating in relation to feelings of:

- **anger**
- **anxiety**
- **boredom**
- **confidence**
- **enthusiasm**
- **fear**
- **frustration**
- **happiness**
- **loneliness**
- **relaxation**
- **stress**
- **tiredness.**

After a bit of number crunching you can be rated on your levels of 'emotional eating', 'restrained eating' (for example, a dieter would tend to fit this category) and 'externalised eating' for example where external factors such as smell affect your eating over internal cues. While tests like these can offer insight, it's good to remember that all constructs such as these have limitations and are never 100 per cent accurate.

Stress clearly affects us all differently. It appears that emotional eaters (those who find comfort in eating when stressed) may in fact be more susceptible to stress and tend to be people who find dietary restraint more challenging. It may be that in the latter case, when faced with a taxing situation or decision, individuals who use dietary restraint to moderate their intake may be distracted by the task at hand and hence their dietary restraint or monitoring is impaired. This is thought to be quite separate from any emotional involvement.

Studies using data from emotional eating scales studies report that low emotional eaters eat less food when they are sad or stressed than high emotional eaters. It also appears (though the results are a little inconsistent) that if you are an emotional eater, during periods of emotional turmoil or stress you will tend to go for high fat, high sugar foods. During times of stress many of us are put right off eating; stress tends to turn off our stomach, releasing sugars into the bloodstream for energy which suppresses feelings of hunger. However, it seems that high emotional eaters don't experience the same response to stress, showing little or no reduction in hunger. In other words, something inside us has changed and, rather than responding innately as our bodies normally would to stress or sadness, something has overwritten this. It is possible that the normal 'fight or flight' response to stress isn't controlled in the same fashion for emotional eaters and, instead of rallying the troops to fight or run, emotional eaters keep on eating.[2]

Cast your mind back to the study by the Australian Psychological Society (p. 111) regarding the critical stage for success when changing eating habits. The same study also looked at the participants in terms of how they cope with emotional challenges and it showed that:

■ **Generally, those who were obese showed lower coping strategies in order to achieve their health goals in the face of stress.**

■ **Obese individuals (and to a lesser degree overweight people in the study) also demonstrated more negative emotions during their attempts at change.**

■ **Obese people in the group also reported the lowest ratings for self-esteem when changing their behaviours to both eating and physical activity.**

■ Interestingly, the study also looked at the importance of physical activity, and while the obese individuals reported the highest level of health risk at not changing their current *eating* behaviours, it was the 'normal' weight group that perceived the greatest health risk from not changing their *physical* activity behaviours and the obese group the lowest.

Quite clearly the distortions we have relate not only to portion size and intake, but also to our health risks.

For some it seems stress can even stimulate eating, which is thought to be counter-intuitive according to the usual stress response by the body.

Tip: Using a scale to determine your level of emotional eating could highlight your susceptibility to stress-induced eating, and in turn you can mount strategies to create new responses to stress cues. Remember, what you are likely going to need to do is rewrite the pathways in your neural system, and while this might take quite a lot of conscious effort, if you persevere it will become the new norm and you'll soon find this new way of eating (or rather, the original, inherent way) will become quite automatic.

How we become emotional eaters is still hotly debated. Some suggest emotional eating hits in our critical years, such as adolescence, and it's something we learn, perhaps as a coping strategy to stresses in our lives around this time in relation to family or similar issues. Potentially some of us are more prone to emotional eating triggers in life or more vulnerable due to a mix of our environment and genetics. We could have the gene for emotional eating or for traits that increase the likelihood of becoming an emotional eater, but if our environment doesn't trigger these we are unaffected. Thought to be a learnt response, emotional eating may be associated with an inability to cope well with stress, and a lowered ability to read internal cues of hunger and satiety. (Yep, there it is again!)

It's also thought that pleasurable eating reduces the stress response, which in turn reinforces our desire and enjoyment around eating and eating more than we require. Hence we come back to mindful eating so that stress-induced excess weight is reduced.

Personality and weight control

Personality is the complex set of unique psychological qualities that influence our characteristic patterns of behaviour across different situations over time. Note that these behaviours are specific to you and are regarded generally under normal circumstances as being:

- stable across different situations
- stable over time.

Having said that, you will see some shifts during critical periods of development as well as during extreme stress.

Personality: The Big 5

So how can we tell what type of personality we have? Personality testing has been around for many, many years. One of the most common foundations used to assess personality is by grouping our traits and using continuums, that is, a line moving from one extreme to the other. For example, in terms of how outgoing we are we can be anywhere along the line from extremely outgoing to painfully shy or anywhere in between. Once we plot ourselves on the various continuums that group our personality traits we can gain insight into the type of personality we have.

The Big 5 Model identifies five main trait groups, each of which is a continuum that goes from one extreme through a relatively neutral state to the polar opposite. The Big 5 are:

1. *Openness*, which spans being curious through to cautious

2. *Conscientiousness*, which includes being efficient and organised at one end to being easygoing through to careless at the other

3. *Extraversion*, being outgoing and energetic to introverted or quiet and reserved (and ambiverts who are at neither extreme but placed in the middle)

4. *Agreeableness*, encompassing compassionate behaviour through to disagreeable, emotionally detached or cold behaviour

5. *Neuroticism*, being a tendency to worry or be anxious through to showing relevant vulnerability through to a lack of sensitivity or care for the usual societal norms.

The personality traits noted in the Big 5 are often used as the basis for personality testing. It's not an exact science and, of course, there is always going to be a level of error and bias, but at the moment it's the best we have. The use of personality profiles is most effective if done by a qualified professional. Nonetheless, most of us have at least a degree of insight into our own personality, and understanding it may allow us to:

- **identify if we are at risk and need assistance**
- **create our own programs tailored to our individual needs as opposed to a 'one size fits all' approach**
- **increase our self-awareness so we can be empowered to create and maintain change for long-term health.**

How does your personality affect your eating?

We need to progress through this minefield carefully; after all, to a degree our personality is set and we can really only tweak the edges of what makes us who we are and reinforce the positives. Please do not use the following information to view yourself in a negative way. Rather, take the positives to work with and view the less desirable aspects as areas to work on.

A great deal of research has been conducted in the area of weight and personality, and in short it seems that certain personality characteristics or traits are associated with being underweight, overweight or obese. For example, it appears that those with issues in maintaining a minimum weight tend to rate higher on what's termed 'neuroticism' scales (for example, they are more prone to phobic or fearful personality traits), while obese individuals tend to rate low on scores of conscientiousness (efforts directed toward specific tasks).

It appears that traits such as impulsivity are positively correlated to our body mass index (BMI) and abdominal girth, so as an individual's impulsivity rating increases so too does their BMI. A large-scale study found that those who tend to worry needlessly (high on neuroticism) and, for whatever reason, evade doing things they don't feel up to (low on conscientiousness), are most vulnerable to gaining unhealthy weight. Add to this another dimension of increased impulsivity and lowered self-discipline and it seems even more likely our waistline will be out of the acceptable range. The study found that people with this set of traits were more likely to give in to temptation and give up.

Logically, to be healthy we must eat healthily and move, and now the research boosts the notion that both of these require commitment and restraint. However, this is a very short-sighted notion: restraint of its own volition brings with it many issues which may work against maintaining a healthy weight. Furthermore, both restraint and commitment will vary from one individual to another regardless of their body shape. And commitment itself requires a full and thorough analysis of habits and how they can be reshaped. Without framing suggestions for ideal personality factors for health within an individual's own context, they can be confusing at best and detrimental at worst. Let's face it, just because you are lean doesn't mean you are conscientious about your eating. It is more likely that you are tuned in to the innate eating habits that work for you.

For those who feel that restrained eating has worked it seems they tend to have traits associated with conscientiousness and achievement, as well as being more outgoing and having stable emotional responses (being less prone to moods, fears, anxiety and so on).[3] Other studies suggest that 'self-control' has little influence on weight control, but as we have discussed there are many more internal and external factors that influence food intake and regulation, many of which may well override or take higher order over personality.[4]

At the end of the day, results regarding which personality traits are involved in weight gain, weight loss and ability to stick with a program differ across each and also sometimes between genders. One trait may be shown to be useful in weight loss but not in sticking with a program. It's just not that simple to say that a certain type of person will be less likely to be overweight and certain personality traits are more beneficial in healthy weight maintenance. The fact is that if we are eating without thought and experiencing the consequences of it we must face this and move forward with positive strategies. As yet there isn't a great deal of work being done on personality and a non-diet approach so we need to keep an open mind when we read material on this topic.

> **Tip:** Focusing on healthy eating, your hunger and satiety cues, and cultivating a positive approach to food is more beneficial than worrying about how your personality affects your weight-loss efforts.

Motivation and weight control

There are many factors in our life that act as driving forces behind our behaviour. Factors that direct and energise our behaviour can be said to be part of what motivates (derived from a Latin word meaning 'to move') us to act. Motivation is a general term for all the processes involved in starting, directing and maintaining physical and psychological activities. Our motivation is affected by our needs, expectations, goals, personality and life experiences.

Studies that have compared obese and non-overweight children's effort to access food found that overweight children are motivated more by food and to consume more energy-dense food and beverages (at least in laboratory settings) than non-overweight children, with the latter children giving up more easily.[5] So it seems the motivation to consume foods is more malleable than our liking. Something that comes up over and over in the research is that motivation to obtain food correlates to our body mass index (BMI) and energy intake more than to our actual liking of a food. Clearly, motivation is an influential factor in our eating habits.

There are three key elements to motivation:

1. Intensity — how much effort is given to a task.

2. Direction — where the effort is directed, its focus.

3. Persistence — how long the effort can be sustained.

Many factors alter our behaviour, for example:

■ **what we expect to occur as a result of our behaviour (or non-behaviour)**

■ **the experiences we have had in the past**

■ **the social and sociological influences in our lives (culture, family, education and groups they belong to)**

■ **the unfulfilled needs that drive us**

■ **our internal states (nervous system activity).**

We have already seen that effort exerts considerable effect over eating. It's important to keep in mind that eating has an automatic element to it as we know, which to some extent can override or counteract these motivational issues. Still, while theories on eating behaviour are not concrete it's important to at least be mindful of the effect of motivation on eating as well as dietary changes.

The relevance of the locus of control

One of the most relevant motivation theories applicable to most aspects of behaviour is the Locus of Control (LOC) by Rotter.[6] The locus of control is a psychological measure that refers to an individual's belief about whether they are personally in control of what happens to them or if they believe external factors beyond their control are. It's a theory that has stood the test of time and one we can all apply to ourselves and see clearly where our motivation lies.

The locus of control relates to what we attribute the outcomes in our lives to (for example, effort or luck). Intrinsic rewards (such as a feeling of improved skills) and extrinsic motivators (rewards) can often be confused with the locus of control — motivators are factors that influence our behaviour, whereas the locus of control is our *belief* about what controls our lives.

A twenty-year follow-up study in the United Kingdom found that adults who as children had a stronger self-belief (higher internal locus of control) had lowered risk of obesity, being overweight, and psychological distress and better self-reports of health, and were more likely to engage in physical activity.[7] In addition, a strong sense of control has been shown to assist in the ongoing maintenance of healthy dietary behaviours in general.

Tip: It is highly likely we can all benefit from harnessing an internal locus of control and recognising the situations where we defer to an external LOC and compromise ourselves.

Internal and external LOC

Rotter's Locus of Control theory suggests that we can attribute outcomes of success and failure in two ways:

- **internally — the belief that our own behaviour influences outcomes, or**
- **externally — the belief that outcomes are attributable to outside factors, for example, luck.**

Here's a quick example. A person who has lost weight might attribute this to the exercise they have undertaken (internal) or to their personal trainer's efforts (external).

In some situations we might attribute the outcome to internal factors and in others to external factors. Often a pattern will emerge regarding the situations we feel most confident in — social, work, sporting, etc. An internal locus of control is closely associated with our self-confidence in a particular situation. For example, at work a person might attribute their successes to luck (external factor) yet in their sporting life they might attribute their failures to a lack of skill (internal factor). Starting to get the picture?

Here are some more general examples highlighting the difference between an internal and external locus of control. Characteristics of a person with an internal locus of control might include:

- **persists in the face of failure**
- **works at tasks for long periods of time**
- **copes well with stress**
- **less susceptible to anxiety**
- **welcomes new challenges**

- actively seeks information about events that affect them

- takes action to improve and overcome shortcomings

- tends to be consistent at school and in other areas of achievement

- sees themselves as being active, powerful, independent and in control of their lives

- takes responsibility for their lives

- experiences success often

- interested in sociopolitical issues

- more likely to see tasks through to completion.

Examples of statements that reflect an internal LOC for losing weight or changing eating habits might include:

- 'I worked really hard to get to this point.'

- 'I put up my plan and referred to it each day.'

- 'I started small and kept it realistic.'

- 'I am really proud of myself with what I have achieved.'

- 'If I didn't understand something I asked.'

- 'I encouraged the rest of my family to join in and help me.'

- 'I changed my work–life balance so I wasn't so stressed.'

If we were to change some of the above statements by using the word 'we' or 'you', you could see that the blame game and deferring begins! Those with an internal locus of control take responsibility for their own situation (as much as it is relevant).

Characteristics of a person with an external locus of control might include:

- **tends to give up in the face of failure**
- **less persistent at tasks**
- **does not cope well with stress**
- **may be susceptible to anxiety**
- **avoids new challenges and change**
- **does not feel the need to seek information about events that affect them (believes other factors control the outcomes)**
- **feels unable to improve and overcome shortcomings**
- **tends to be inconsistent at school and in other areas of achievement**
- **sees themself as being passive, powerless, dependent and not in control of their lives**
- **tends not to take responsibility for their life**
- **feels the experience of success is rare**
- **uninterested in sociopolitical issues**
- **less likely to see tasks through to completion.**

Examples of statements that reflect an external LOC for losing weight or changing eating habits could include:

- **'Diets never work for me.'**
- **'No diet has ever worked for me.'**
- **'I have tried everything.'**

- 'You didn't help much.'

- 'We don't eat like that in our family.'

- 'I am afraid of being hungry.'

- 'I am afraid if I try I will fail.'

- 'I can't exercise as I am too big/unfit/puffed/sore.'

- 'My mother was big so I will be big too.'

- 'Genetically my family are all big so I will be too.'

- 'I am too old to change.'

- 'I can't cook.'

- 'I don't know what to buy.'

- 'I am too busy to exercise.'

- 'It's too embarrassing to exercise.'

Emotional response to experiences by locus of control

How we respond to outcomes can give a strong indication of our locus of control. For example, if I am supposed to walk the dog three days a week but never get around to it and report feeling guilty, then I am acknowledging my role in the failure and this is an internal locus of control. Having said that, the action I take to remedy this is important!

The emotional impact of our locus of control varies with the locus and with the outcome. This is highlighted opposite in Table 8.

Table 8: Emotional responses to experiences by LOC

Individuals with an internal LOC who experience:	Individuals with an external LOC who experience:
1. SUCCESS tend to feel pride confidence competence satisfaction	**1. SUCCESS may feel** gratitude thankfulness luck
2. FAILURE tend to feel guilt shame incompetence depression	**2. FAILURE may feel** anger surprise astonishment

Being able to recognise these emotional responses, and consider our locus of control, can provide a means to motivate us. For example, we might attribute a successful outcome to a friend despite the active role we have played. When we recognise this we can reflect on the role we played in our success and consolidate our self-recognition (enhancing an internal locus of control).

How to develop an internal locus of control

Self-confidence should be fostered; for example, in sport winners tend to attribute outcomes to internal, non-changing (stable) and controllable causes. The following are suggestions to strengthen self-confidence:

- Be encouraged to attribute outcomes to internal causes (for example, training and effort) when appropriate.

- Try to attribute your failure to unstable (changeable) causes such as effort. Giving reasons that are stable (for example, ability) may cause a lack of confidence.

- Reasons for success should be stable (such as ability) which encourages self-confidence.

In many ways you could view this simply as focusing on the things you can change for the better and working with your strong points!

Improving internal LOC

Below is a list of ways for improving your internal locus of control. Changing your LOC is not something that occurs either easily or quickly; it is best achieved via slow and continual monitoring.

- Assume responsibility for tasks that you must accomplish — offer to do tasks you would not normally undertake, initially ensuring that they are not too difficult.

- Try new tasks over the ones you have always done — alter your experience of your life and be open to new and positive ways of doing things.

- Challenge your habits — look at the areas of your life (friends, work, sport) and your own beliefs and values and reassess any that reinforce your external locus of control.

Healthful eating task:
Recognising LOC statements

The aim here is to become familiar with LOC statements so you will be able to recognise them in yourself and in others.

Task 1: The following are statements made by an individual with an external locus of control. Re-write the statements below, wording each in a way that an individual with an internal locus of control would make them (the first one is done for you).

1. My family doesn't like healthy food, so it is too hard to change what I eat.

2. Diets never work for me.

3. I have tried everything and nothing works for me.

4. I can't exercise, I am too big.

5. Maybe I could lose weight if we bought better food when we went grocery shopping.

Answers

1. *I have not been able to change my family eating habits and that is affecting my weight goals.*

2.

3.

4.

5.

Task 2: *Determine if the statements below are examples of an internal locus of control or an external locus of control. Circle 'internal' or 'external' for each.*

1. I have kept the weight off for seven months because I learnt that the first six months are critical so I joined a group to keep me on track.
internal / external

2. I have managed to keep the weight off for seven months because my friend pushed me.
internal / external

3. I have been able to eat more of a variety of vegetables because I have stocked the cupboards and attended a cooking class.
internal / external

4. I am eating better because my girlfriend has been cooking healthy meals for me.
internal / external

7
Media
and
marketing

We all sing along to various jingles and laugh over other advertisements. But do we follow advertising and marketing trends or are they following us? Who is really creating the trends? Are we just sheep and following the leader? Or are our deepest desires simply being used against us? After all, don't most of us buy things we really don't need based on some sort of precipitated desire to live life how the adverts portray it?

Let's take a look at just how powerful even subtle advertising is on our buying habits. The beauty in doing this is that it brings to our conscious mind many unconscious forces that can direct our food choices; this way, we can ensure that the dog is wagging the tail, and not the other way around, ideally creating a transparent and level playing ground for us all.

It's not all bad. There are some who are 'marketing' to us for non-commercial reasons, for example health departments educating us about excessive salt intake or the health effects of alcohol and so on. Information about consumers provides valuable insight into how to not only sell products for the bottom line, but how to encourage healthy eating and healthy lifestyles.

Where do you belong in the marketplace?

You may not like being referred to as being part of a market segmentation, but if you spend your hard-earned money you will be analysed into a consumer subgroup according to many of your personal factors such as where you live, what you spend your money on, your demographics (income, employment, age, gender, etc.), psychological needs and motivation, cultural factors and so on. Market segments influence how best to market a product.

Your values are valuable!

In psychology it's well established that to create behavioural change a person's habits must be clearly defined. In order to sell salad in a fast food outlet, marketing campaigns must be clear on what will drive a person to purchase such a food from such an outlet.

Psychographic segmentation is based on our values, attitudes and lifestyles, and is commonly referred to as VALS. VALS was originally devised in the United States in the 1970s, with the creation of the VALS Framework (see Figure 8 opposite).

Figure 8:
The VALS framework[1]

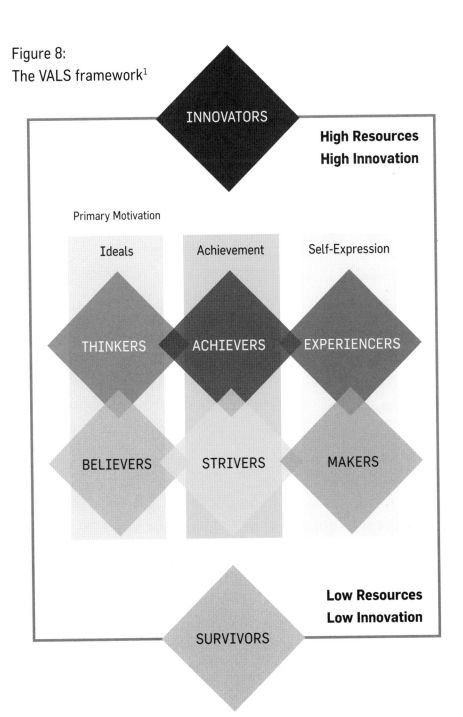

'So,' you might say, 'that's all very interesting but how does that affect what we eat?' At a broader level we can see that this model is based on two basic market segments:

- **INNOVATORS who have a lot of resources at their disposal, such as income, and**
- **SURVIVORS who have low resources at their disposal.**

Divided between this continuum are six groups:

- **Thinkers**
- **Achievers**
- **Experiencers**
- **Believers**
- **Strivers**
- **Makers.**

Table 9 on p. 160 gives you a fuller description of these groups. Spend a moment and consider where you sit. Which group do you belong to in relation to your food shopping habits? How about your boss? What about your parents? It's likely that each will differ and your motives to purchase certain foods over others is driven by different things.

Beginning to see the logic? Great! As we can see, resources that are likely to be available to each act as drivers or motivators that encourage each group's consumer behaviours. Let's take, for example, the Experiencers. They are impulsive and believe in self-expression, compared to Survivors who are focused on basic needs and not generally interested in 'fancy' things.

Does marketing matter?

If you had any doubt that marketing is a powerful influence on our spending and consumption habits, consider the following facts that might convince you of its impact.

- For every $1 the World Health Organization (WHO) spends on initiatives to better the nutrition of the world's population, the food industry spends $500 promoting processed food.[2]

- The food, drink and confectionery industries spent US$13 billion on worldwide advertising in 2006.[3]

- In Australia, McDonald's is reported to have spent AU$90,000 on a 30-second TV advertisement of one of its new burgers plus a AU$10 million product launch. Now, $90,000 may not sound like much but the advert ran for just three days, and it's estimated that Australians spent AU$2 million in one week on the product. In total the product is believed to have doubled its projected sales in the first month alone.[4]

Table 9: Descriptions of consumer segments

Segment	Description
Psychographic segmentation based on values	*Attitudes and lifestyles (VALS) as devised in the US in the 1970s.*
Innovators	High disposable income, enjoy change, they're independent and like the 'finer things in life.'
Thinkers	Mature tastes, reflective thinkers, often conservative with some respect for status quo but also some healthy scepticism.
Achievers	Conventional lives, image is important, tend toward established prestige.
Experiencers	Generally young, thrill-seekers, with impulsive buying behaviour.
Believers	Conservative, brand loyal and conventional.
Strivers	Impulsive buyers often following trends.
Makers	Older, more traditional consumers, respect for bureaucracy, hard working.
Survivors	Linear lifestyle, focused on daily needs.

Resources	Drives
With the creation of the VALS Framework.	*Psychographic segmentation based on values.*
Have easy access to resources.	Self image, status and reflecting financial success.
Easy access and often well educated and can critique well.	Ideals, value, functionality.
Commitment to career and success; value consensus.	Image, goals, success.
Good income and tend to spend a lot of it.	Self-expression, activity, fitting in.
Strong conservative beliefs and philosophies.	Ideals and familiarity.
Not as much access as they would wish.	Achievement, views of others, often follow 'heroes'.
Skills and conviction.	Value as opposed to luxury.
Limited access.	Basic needs.

Healthful eating task:
Increase your awareness of marketing

This task will help you distinguish between the different consumer segments and become more aware of how marketing and advertising utilise shopping data.

Consider each of the products below. Next to each product, write in the consumer you think would be most motivated to purchase it (for example, Experiencers, Makers, etc.). Keep in mind that some products might be used by two or more consumer groups so your answers may differ from ours.

Product	Answer
Brand-name cereal	
Large brand-name pure fruit juice with small juice free	
Heat-neutral juice extractor that retains enzymes	
Locally grown mangoes	
iPhone recipe app	
Swiss chocolate or French sparkling water	
Salt-reduced Heinz Baked Beans	
Organic chocolate-covered goji berries	

Take yourself out of the market(ing)

Marketing works on factors that relate to the product itself such as its taste, packaging and price, which are called intrinsic factors; and extrinsic factors, which are external to the product and include features such as shelf placement and promotions.

In broad terms, marketing is based on the four Ps.

- **PRODUCT:** an intrinsic factor, includes characteristics of the product such as the taste, smell, look and even packaging and labelling that appeals to consumers.

- **PRICE:** also an intrinsic factor, ensures that the product is appealing to the demographic of the market by setting the appropriate price point — too cheap and it can 'dilute' the brand's appeal, too expensive and it can price its main consumer out of the market.

- **PLACE:** an extrinsic cue, which includes the location of the product on the shelf, the store it is sold in and so on.

- **PROMOTION:** an extrinsic factor including how often the product is seen, what it is promoted in conjunction with, who promotes it and the message that is used.

Let's consider advertising and its goals.

- **To enhance brand loyalty,** in other words to encourage us to stick with their brand over others.

- **To increase the number of brand-loyal consumers,** that is to get those using other products to switch.

- **To gain new brand-loyal customers, that is, to gain not just those already using a similar product but those who have never used the product or service before (a good example would be a child).**

Advertisers can appeal to us directly, for example, by using facts — we are all familiar with campaigns encouraging smokers to cut back on smoking. They can also appeal to us indirectly, for example, using impressions of a lifestyle to sell a car. The indirect (also referred to as the peripheral) route is based on the assumption that our feelings and what we identify with are important in our decision-making processes, in fact potentially they have a stronger effect than our logical processing side.

In terms of food advertising, peripheral adverts appear to work on us by directly accessing many of our behaviours. It seems that such emotive adverts that appeal to who we are or how we want our lives to be, are more persuasive than adverts presenting facts.[5] Fact-based adverts tap into our reasoning, eliciting us to use logical rules. This process is time-consuming and deliberate. Hence, direct advertising can require us to enlist a far greater degree of processing, unlike the peripheral adverts that appeal more to intuitive processing which is much faster and more automatic. As such, indirect means of advertising tend to use images, feelings, symbols and implied messages to get us into a buying frenzy.

Healthful eating task: Pay attention to advertising

Tonight as you watch TV, pause for a moment after an advert that has created a strong feeling in you, perhaps a dreamy state of 'If only life was really like that'. Ask yourself what emotions this advert sparked in you. Simply being consciously aware of these sorts of factors can change how you feel about a product.

The importance of branding to product success

Branding is the strategy used to create and influence consumers' brand preferences, in other words our buying behaviour. Branding is used to create a perception of a product that in many cases is aimed at initiating an emotional tie to the product, the brand or the company. Keep in mind the difference between a brand and a company. For example, Cornflakes is the brand and the company is Kellogg's; similarly, KitKat is the brand and Nestlé is the company.

It has been shown that brand perceptions (impressions of a brand) can influence buying behaviour. For example, successful branding can:

- **create a justification for us to pay more for that product than for other brands**
- **create a loyalty towards that product or company over others**
- **elicit a positive emotional view of the product or company and strengthen the above effects.**

Branding has a strong affect on many consumers. One study showed that simply wrapping a food in a McDonald's wrapper can increase the liking of that food (by individuals who like such food).[6] Likewise the total amount consumed of the branded product tends to increase under such conditions. Advertisements can affect our choices, preferences, liking and intake and children appear particularly susceptible to branding and advertising.

The effect of advertising on eating

This is probably no surprise to you but it seems that advertising of food has a direct causal link to us consuming greater amounts of snacks. While the advertisers might try to suggest that advertising affects only brand loyalty and preferences and not nutrition, studies in the area suggest otherwise.[7] But wait, there's more! Our level of hunger (in both children and adults) before this effect takes hold doesn't appear to influence this overconsumption; in fact, the effect is such that even if you are not consuming food at the time of exposure to an advert it can still increase the amount you eat at a later meal, hence the concern regarding advertising and excessive intake of food. You could be forgiven for feeling that the advertisers are working against our good health.

While many countries have introduced self-regulatory measures at an industry level, most of these have fairly narrow scope and there are ongoing issues around the effectiveness of self-regulation.

Tip: Just turning off the TV around meal times can go a long way towards helping you change eating habits for the better.

Who is sending us healthy messages?

In Australia, the most commonly advertised food in magazines offering health messages is in fact processed foods (which are generally less nutritionally sound options). Studies have found that most healthy eating messages in such magazines are provided by manufacturers, at double the rate of retailers. Sadly, non-commercial sources of healthy eating information represent just 2 per cent.[8]

Research in the United States in 2007 found that just over half of the top marketed children's foods which included fruit on their packaging actually contained (yes, you guessed it) no fruit at all.[9] Still in the United States, in 2012 fast food outlets 'forked out' a sum of US$4.6 billion on advertising. Just to put this into context, McDonald's, who had the largest advertising budget, spent almost three times the amount spent in the United States on all fruit, vegies, bottled water and milk advertising, and that's combined.[10] And as if that's not enough to convince you, US fast food outlets loaded 6 billion ads onto Facebook in 2012, which is said to represent just under 20 per cent of all their online advertising![11]

Tip: Shop according to your health needs, try to tune out to food advertising, don't watch TV around dinner and supper times, and focus on your personal health goals.

8
Food labelling

Placing nutritional information on packaging is a popular endeavour today, but you have to ask, 'Just how much information can you fit on a packet before it simply becomes a confusing mural?' GI ratings, percentages of RDI, DIs, RIs, ticks, logos, low this and high that, the list goes on. However, while the nutrition panel may be intimidating, it can provide you with some simple information that is both relevant and reliable.

Nutrition panels

The nutrition panel on a food product can provide you with information on energy (in calories or kilojoules), serving size, the number of servings in the product, carbohydrates and sugars, fat and saturated fat, protein, fibre and sodium (salt). This information is often given for both a serving size and 100g, at least in countries such as the United Kingdom, Australia and New Zealand. A list of ingredients will also be included, which can be very useful when trying to avoid, for example, products that contain hidden sugars.

Nutrition panels are definitely your friend! If you have ever found yourself glazing over while scanning a nutrition panel because of the sheer volume of numbers staring back at you, glaze over no longer. There is a real advantage in being able to sift out the important bits. You might be surprised at just how easy it is to use these very handy numbers to pick the best products for you and your family.

Start with the 100g column

You can find up to four columns of information on a nutrition panel in some countries. Trying to interpret all that information for a trolley full of shopping is likely to mean you will have to take your sleeping bag for the trip! To make it simple, just look at the 100g panel where possible. Not only is it easy to read, but it also means that when comparing products you are comparing relevant values. For example, let's say you are comparing two cereals: one product has a serving size of 40g and another has one of 30g. By using the 'per 100g' panel you are comparing 'apples with apples'.

The United States uses a different method of labelling, instead using percentages of daily values. Daily values can be in reference to requirements as well as upper limits — for example, you can check for the daily value of a nutrient (such as iron) you need sufficient levels of in your diet for health, or you can check if you are exceeding a nutrient you need to limit (such as salt).

But what about the other columns?

Using the 'per serve' column is good to give you an idea of the amount of a nutrient that just one standard serve (as deemed by the manufacturer) of the product will contribute overall. In some cases you will also find a DI or 'total daily intake' (Australia and NZ) and RIs (reference intakes) in the United Kingdom or DVs (daily values) in the United States. Such figures represent the approximate amount (and the actual reference amount of, for example, total calories differs from one country to another), often shown in percentages, of a nutrient or of energy required for health. The reference amount is a standard figure based on an average person. Keep in mind that servings may be less relevant for a food you would eat with other foods, and also what a manufacturer considers a serve might differ from what you would eat in a sitting.

Carbs and sugars — know the difference!

Now here is a great piece of consumer power! By using the carbohydrate and sugars figures you can find products with less simple sugar. This can be a great way of improving fibre and more complex forms of carbohydrates in your diet and keeping simple sugars in balance.

Here's how you do it. Consider the following.

- The *total carbohydrates* figure represents all sugars, naturally occurring and added, simple and complex.

- The *total sugars* figure, on the other hand, indicates how much of these carbohydrates are simple sugars (naturally occurring and added).

It's important to point out that not all simple sugars are bad; in fact, naturally occurring ones such as lactose from milk and fructose from fruit have many health functions. Added sugar is the 'bad guy', with more and more studies showing how it contributes to weight issues, diabetes and even cancer.

Tip: **Remember, when a diet demonises a naturally occurring nutrient like fat or sugar, you have to think carefully about that diet's merits as we have already seen.**

While these figures don't tell you if the sugars are added (that's where the ingredients panel is best), it will show you what proportion of the carbohydrates are simple sugars, and what proportion come from more complex carbohydrates that are associated with many health benefits.

Other columns

You may also see a column listing 'Quantity per serving' when the product is eaten in conjunction with other foods — for example, a breakfast cereal nutrition panel might show a nutrient breakdown column with milk.

Cutting the fat in the numbers

Recent findings from Europe have questioned the low-fat era.[1] In reality, it may make more sense to eat food as it is intended. For example, if a food is predominantly unhealthy saturated fats and/or trans fat then logically such food should be consumed in conservative amounts. Unfortunately many fat-altered products are often high in sugar and/or salt. As we are now finding, added sugar has the potential to do as much damage to our health as unhealthy saturated fats and trans fat, and excessive salt isn't too far behind in those stakes.

It's important to point out here that labelling of trans fat in foods differs from one country to the next and, in fact, can change at any given time. In the United States the FDA requires trans fats to be listed on food labels. In Australia and New Zealand the tide continues to shift — as of late 2013 Food Standards Australia NZ do not require mandatory labelling unless the manufacturer makes a claim in reference to fats on their label. The United Kingdom and Europe generally also have no mandatory requirement for trans fat labelling and hence the British Dietetics Association recommends that you read labels carefully for the presence of partially hydrogenated fats, suggesting that the further up the ingredients list the more likely the product is to have higher levels of trans fats.[2]

You are not going to be bombarded with percentages of fats here and there. Rather, let's return to just good old informed personal choice and common sense. Here are a few tips to consider if you are concerned about fat.

- Focus on good fats such as those found in nuts and seeds, fish, avocado, etc., and simply cut back on products you know to have a lot of unhealthy saturated fats and/or trans fats. Remember, whole foods are better in most cases than processed foods.

- Animal products (excluding fish) will be higher in saturated fat (that's why you don't see overweight plants) and hence should be eaten in moderate amounts.

- Watch out for claims about cholesterol. Plant foods don't contain cholesterol, so to say that chips are cooked in cholesterol-free vegetable oil could be a little misleading.

- Also, cholesterol in food and the cholesterol our body makes (in response to the fat we eat) do very different things in our body, with the latter being the one to watch out for. So don't be misled by cholesterol content in food — it's the bad fat you eat that causes cholesterol issues, that is, trans fats. Cholesterol made by our body is used for our hormone production and so on.

■ Avoid foods with partially hydrogenated fats and oils.

■ 'Low fat' doesn't necessarily equate to healthy. Check your fat-altered products for other 'tasty' ingredients such as sugar and salt or simply use the unaltered product in minimal amounts.

However, food is much more than just a few nutrients — there are hundreds of vitamins, minerals and health compounds we require for good health. And let's not forget that eating should be about more than just numbers; it's about quality ingredients and enjoyable foods that add variety to our diet and nourish our bodies.

We see nutrition information everywhere today, even in our restaurants and at fast-food joints. But has this really helped? Is this simply preaching to the converted and being ignored by those who could perhaps benefit? Are we overloaded with so much information that it's all white noise now? Do we really need to be told that something barely resembling its origins might have lost some of its benefits?

Food labels: do they have an effect?

The degree to which food labels actually drive behaviour is as yet not entirely understood. However, studies show that we don't fully utilise the information on packaging nor do we entirely understand the message, particularly where there is an analytical requirement (maths isn't everyone's favourite thing to do while grocery shopping). In order for labels to drive consumer choice, we must better define target groups and relevant methods of learning and translate this into labelling codes.

Studies also show that the size of information displayed, colour schemes and our familiarity with positioning all affect what consumers pay attention to on a label.[3]

So, clearly labels can have an effect; the question is how to ensure this is a positive one. Here's a question for you to consider: does the mere fact that we need food labels to tell us if a food is a healthy option the actual issue? One could suggest that if we ate based on healthy eating principles — that is, if we ate a diet high in a variety of unprocessed, whole foods that suits our individual needs — we wouldn't really need all those labels on such foods. Is healthy eating really only achievable if we are told what to eat, or is it something that becomes more intuitive? The more complex we make something so simple, the further away we seem to get from our goal. Just a thought!

Packaging messages

Manufacturers have a number of ways in which they can influence our food selection, this includes the use of descriptive names on menus or packaging, the mention of certain ingredients or meal attributes, or calorie labelling on restaurant menus. There is substantial evidence of the impact health claims on packaging have on food choice.

Given the apparent lack of real understanding gained from labels and the 'room' the industry has for disseminating information, what is said and presented must be carefully controlled. You could liken it to teaching a child to learn to read: you don't launch into *Harry Potter* at age four or five, as clearly at this age a child's understanding of many of the concepts and even phrases in such books would be limited. Likewise, marketing shouldn't be allowed to effect considerable control over the susceptible, and nor should it be able to misrepresent products to the unaware. Even some nutritionists find decoding products challenging!

Health claims

Codex Alimentarius is one of the major organisations in relation to health claim guidelines. They note that in essence there are three types of health claims made by companies or food producers about their products.

- **Nutrient function claims: in other words claims that describe a nutrient and its role in growth, development and health, for example, vitamin B6 is used in energy production.**

- **Functional claims: these relate to how a nutrient or compound affects body function, for example, that protein helps to grow strong bodies.**

- **Reduced risk of disease or illness claims: for example, that folic acid reduces neural tube defects in developing foetuses.**

Interestingly, studies suggest that while we are influenced by health claims to the point where we will be more inclined to purchase positively viewed products, we still view them with scepticism and agree that government regulation is required. Few consumers are able to discern the difference between functional claims and nutrient claims and as such find them confusing, with a preference for short, relevant wording where claims are used.[4]

The example of sodium

The Australian Division of World Action on Salt and Health found that consumers considered salt the third leading nutrient of concern (after saturated fat and sugar, and interestingly both of these nutrients were demonised incorrectly).[5] Yet recent data suggests that food industry symbols on packaging don't assist us in selecting low sodium foods. Interestingly, Australians seem to be aware that processed foods contribute significantly to excessive dietary salt, though the two biggest contributors in the Australian diet, bread and breakfast cereals, were not generally viewed as major contributors to salt intake. Yes, that's right, compare the sodium level of your favourite bread next time you grab a loaf and you'll find that the low sodium range of 120mg per 100g in Australia and 1.5g of salt per 100g in the United Kingdom is not even close when it comes to some commercial bread!

In the United Kingdom around 8.1g of salt is consumed every day — that's just under two teaspoons and about 2g more than is recommended by UK authorities. Again, around 75 per cent of the salt in the UK diet comes from premade foods we purchase, such as processed meats, crisps, breads, pasta sauces, other sauces for meals, soups, breakfast cereals and of course the old favourite crisps! In the United Kingdom, a high range for salt in a food is considered 1.5g of salt or more per 100g of product (this equates to 0.6g of sodium), while a low-salt food is considered that which has 0.3g per 100g or 0.1g of sodium per 100g. In the United States, low sodium products are said to be those with 140mg or less per serving.

While most of us understand the health implication of excessive salt, the numbers of us opting for a low-salt diet just don't match. Studies reveal that almost 70 per cent of us report we review the nutrition panel regarding sodium; this is largely done by those of us who believe lowering salt in our diet will assist with our health. One in three of us may regularly purchase 'low-salt' or 'no added salt' products, yet many are unable to determine what constitutes a low-salt product or tell the difference between sodium and salt (a combination of sodium and chloride.).

Logos and endorsements on food products

An increasing number of logos, symbols and even famous faces are appearing on food product labels or in adverts for them, providing additional information and at the same time potentially more confusing information for consumers. Logos and personalities can have a powerful impact on our buying habits, but it's worth keeping in mind that even though someone endorses a product it doesn't mean they use it themselves.

Well-known logos include those showing a product's GI (glycaemic index) as well as certifications from heart associations, which will vary from country to country (some examples include Australia's Heart Foundation Tick and the US Heart-Check mark). Two important considerations should be noted: firstly that most consumers are unaware of the actual criteria used in the certification process (though much of it is available). And secondly, just because a product doesn't have an endorsement of this sort doesn't mean it is necessarily in any way inferior to those that do. Consumer groups point out that such promotions may also give the impression that foods with endorsements can be consumed in greater quantities, sometimes at the expense of whole foods such as fruit and vegetables that have been shown to have many health-giving benefits. Ultimately you are likely to find that if you read the ingredients panel and nutrition panel you can make a pretty good assessment of the product yourself.

Simple tips for choosing products

Let's be sensible about eating. There was an advertisement in New Zealand some years back where a young girl asks her mum what the difference is between butter and margarine, to which her mum replies, 'Ask your dad, he's the chemist.' Real people eat real food!

At a quick glance you'll be able to determine a product's nutritional offerings from the following simple tips.

- Increase fresh food and cut back on processed. Ta-daa! No labels to read and a whole lot healthier too.

- Quickly review the ingredients panel for the presence of sugar and other simple sugars such as honey, sucrose, maltose, etc.

- Avoid/limit products where sugar is high up on the ingredients list or where there are multiple added sugars.

- Knowing how many kilojoules or calories are in a product doesn't necessarily give you an indication of the quality and wholesomeness of the product. Opt for foods that have whole foods over processed ones in the ingredients — this is more likely to increase the nutritional benefits and lower the unwanted compounds or excesses.

- Focus on quality not numbers, particularly when you are choosing products for children who should not be on restricted diets unless under the supervision of a qualified health professional.

- Opt for products that resemble their starting ingredients. For example, whole-bean soy drinks, wholegrain bread. Opt for whole foods, real meat, real fruit, vegies and yoghurt, cold-pressed oils, homemade sauces and spreads and so on. This step is very likely to reduce exposure to additives, trans and unhealthy saturated fats, added sugar and salt, as well as increase the nutrients you gain.

9
Making
changes

Congratulations, you've made it! That's a lot of information to take in and a lot of ideas to consider. You now need to decide which of that information you'll take action on. So where do you start?

Importantly, keep it simple. Potentially one of the areas that will afford you the greatest benefits is re-sensitising yourself to your internal cues of hunger and fullness. Ask yourself how hungry you are before you eat and how much you should eat based on this. Then, after you have eaten a relevant portion size, ask yourself how full you are and if you need to continue to eat or not. Do this for just one month or at least until it begins to become second nature again, until you have reshaped your eating habits back to your original eating habits when you were young, when you ate what you needed, enjoyed every mouthful and stopped when you were full.

This is best determined by you. There are all the tips and tricks along the way about serving spoon size, food placement, plate size and so on, but just which ones will work for you will depend on you and your life. Set your vision of how you want yourself and your life to be, imagine what that feels like, what you will be doing. Create a whole vision, set your short-term goals and gather the tools that will set you on your course. Work through your goals slowly and from time to time reflect on how you are going — self-evaluation is very important — and focus on your health rather than society-driven views of what you should look like. We all want to be here for as long as we can, for our family and friends, and just importantly we want to be vital throughout our lives, to live well.

Some pointers

1. Set clear goals and ensure you have clear, practical processes to achieve the goal/s

- Goals should be set by you and any others involved and should be relevant to your lifestyle and personal situation rather than an external idealised view.
- Details of how your goals will be achieved need to be documented for transparency as well as direction and evaluation.

2. Break goals down into small, achievable, short-term goals

- Ensure any goals you set are small steps that are achievable, as this will motivate you and encourage commitment.

3. **Include those involved in the changes to the decision-making process**

   ■ If others are going to be involved in your efforts towards healthier eating (family members, for example), include them in any decision making. This will likely improve compliance and success as it provides an opportunity for those involved to 'own' the process.

4. **Be aware of gender and age differences**

   ■ If your family is involved in these changes, consider the effect of the various gender and ages of family members and how this might affect both how healthier eating habits relate to them and the differences with respect to each age group's needs.

5. **Encourage positive self-esteem**

   ■ Ensure you stop to acknowledge the positives, your gains and successes. Explore these to understand what changes and factors have contributed to your improvements.

6. **Challenge societal images of body shapes**

   ■ Look around you and notice just how much pressure we can place upon ourselves when following irrational and unrealistic social norms and images. Challenge this and reinforce your own realistic, positive, health-based goals.

7. **Don't be afraid to challenge old values that limit**

   ■ Question yourself about why something is so and why

it must continue. Questioning is an excellent method of identifying and challenging negative values or self-limiting behaviours.

8. Remember, what we know is very limited and there is much more to learn!

- It has been said that the greatest strength is vulnerability. Humility is a very great quality and recognising that, of all there is to know, we know so very little. This allows you to be open to change and new understanding.

Appendix 1:
Dutch Eating Behaviour Questionnaire[1]

This questionnaire measures your levels of restrained, emotional and external eating. Please answer honestly rather than what you think might be the 'right' answer. Read each question and circle the answer that is true for you.

1. If you have put on weight, do you eat less than you usually do?

Not relevant   *Never*   *Seldom*   *Sometimes*   *Often*   *Very often*

2. Do you try to eat less at mealtimes than you would like to eat?

Never   *Seldom*   *Sometimes*   *Often*   *Very often*

3. How often do you refuse food or drink offered because you are concerned about your weight?

Never   *Seldom*   *Sometimes*   *Often*   *Very often*

4. Do you watch exactly what you eat?

Never   *Seldom*   *Sometimes*   *Often*   *Very often*

5. Do you deliberately eat foods that are slimming?

          Never   *Seldom*   *Sometimes*   *Often*   *Very often*

6. When you have eaten too much, do you eat less than usual on the following days?

Not relevant   *Never*   *Seldom*   *Sometimes*   *Often*   *Very often*

7. Do you deliberately eat less in order not to become heavier?

          Never   *Seldom*   *Sometimes*   *Often*   *Very often*

8. How often do you try not to eat between meals because you are watching your weight?

          Never   *Seldom*   *Sometimes*   *Often*   *Very often*

9. How often in the evening do you try not to eat because you are watching your weight?

          Never   *Seldom*   *Sometimes*   *Often*   *Very often*

10. Do you take into account your weight with what you eat?

          Never   *Seldom*   *Sometimes*   *Often*   *Very often*

11. Do you have a desire to eat when you are irritated?

Not relevant   *Never*   *Seldom*   *Sometimes*   *Often*   *Very often*

12. Do you have a desire to eat when you have nothing to do?

Not relevant   *Never*   *Seldom*   *Sometimes*   *Often*   *Very often*

13. Do you have a desire to eat when you are depressed or discouraged?

Not relevant   Never   Seldom   Sometimes   Often   Very often

14. Do you have a desire to eat when you are feeling lonely?

Not relevant   Never   Seldom   Sometimes   Often   Very often

15. Do you have a desire to eat when somebody lets you down?

Not relevant   Never   Seldom   Sometimes   Often   Very often

16. Do you have a desire to eat when you are cross?

Not relevant   Never   Seldom   Sometimes   Often   Very often

17. Do you have a desire to eat when you are waiting for something unpleasant to happen?

Never   Seldom   Sometimes   Often   Very often

18. Do you get the desire to eat when you are anxious, worried or tense?

Never   Seldom   Sometimes   Often   Very often

19. Do you have a desire to eat when things are going against you or when things have gone wrong?

Never   Seldom   Sometimes   Often   Very often

20. Do you have a desire to eat when you are frightened?

Not relevant   Never   Seldom   Sometimes   Often   Very often

21. Do you have a desire to eat when you are disappointed?

Not relevant   *Never*   *Seldom*   *Sometimes*   *Often*   *Very often*

22. Do you have a desire to eat when you are emotionally upset?

Not relevant   *Never*   *Seldom*   *Sometimes*   *Often*   *Very often*

23. Do you have a desire to eat when you are bored or restless?

Not relevant   *Never*   *Seldom*   *Sometimes*   *Often*   *Very often*

24. If food tastes good to you, do you eat more than usual?

Never   *Seldom*   *Sometimes*   *Often*   *Very often*

25. If food smells and looks good, do you eat more than usual?

Never   *Seldom*   *Sometimes*   *Often*   *Very often*

26. If you see or smell something delicious, do you have a desire to eat it?

Never   *Seldom*   *Sometimes*   *Often*   *Very often*

27. If you have something delicious to eat, do you eat it straightaway?

Never   *Seldom*   *Sometimes*   *Often*   *Very often*

28. If you walk past the bakery do you have the desire to buy something delicious?

Never   *Seldom*   *Sometimes*   *Often*   *Very often*

29. If you walk past a snack bar or a café, do you have the desire to buy something delicious?

Never   Seldom   Sometimes   Often   Very often

30. If you see others eating, do you also have the desire to eat?

Never   Seldom   Sometimes   Often   Very often

31. Can you resist eating delicious foods?

Never   Seldom   Sometimes   Often   Very often

32. Do you eat more than usual when you see others eating?

Never   Seldom   Sometimes   Often   Very often

33. When preparing a meal are you inclined to eat something?

Never   Seldom   Sometimes   Often   Very often

Scoring: Calculate scores for questions 1–10, 11–23 and 24–33 separately. Never = 1, Seldom = 2, Sometimes = 3, Often = 4, Very often = 5, Not relevant = 0.

Add up scores for items 1–10 and divide by 10 for the Restrained eating subscale score.

Add up scores for items 11–23 and divide by 13 for the Emotional eating subscale score.

Add up scores for items 24–33, reversing the score for item 31, and then divide by 10 for the External eating subscale score.

Subscale	Restrained (items 1–10)	Emotional (items 11–23)	External (items 24–33)
Total of scores			(remember to reverse score for item 31)
Divide by	10	13	10
Final subscale score			

Appendix 2:
Intuitive Eating Scale[1]

For each item, please circle the answer that best characterises your attitudes or behaviours.

1. I try to avoid certain foods high in fat, carbohydrates or calories.

Strongly disagree   *Disagree*   *Neutral*   *Agree*   *Strongly agree*

2. I stop eating when I feel full (not overstuffed).

Strongly disagree   *Disagree*   *Neutral*   *Agree*   *Strongly agree*

3. I find myself eating when I'm feeling emotional (for example, anxious, depressed, sad), even when I'm not physically hungry.

Strongly disagree   *Disagree*   *Neutral*   *Agree*   *Strongly agree*

4. If I am craving a certain food, I allow myself to have it.

Strongly disagree   *Disagree*   *Neutral*   *Agree*   *Strongly agree*

5. I follow eating rules or dieting plans that dictate what, when and/ or how much to eat.

Strongly disagree   *Disagree*   *Neutral*   *Agree*   *Strongly agree*

6. I find myself eating when I am bored, even when I'm not physically hungry.

Strongly disagree   *Disagree*   *Neutral*   *Agree*   *Strongly agree*

7. I can tell when I'm slightly full.

Strongly disagree   *Disagree*   *Neutral*   *Agree*   *Strongly agree*

8. I can tell when I'm slightly hungry.

Strongly disagree   *Disagree*   *Neutral*   *Agree*   *Strongly agree*

9. I get mad at myself for eating something unhealthy.

Strongly disagree   *Disagree*   *Neutral*   *Agree*   *Strongly agree*

10. I find myself eating when I am lonely, even when I'm not physically hungry.

Strongly disagree   *Disagree*   *Neutral*   *Agree*   *Strongly agree*

11. I trust my body to tell me when to eat.

Strongly disagree   *Disagree*   *Neutral*   *Agree*   *Strongly agree*

12. I trust my body to tell me what to eat.

Strongly disagree   *Disagree*   *Neutral*   *Agree*   *Strongly agree*

13. I trust my body to tell me how much to eat.

Strongly disagree   *Disagree*   *Neutral*   *Agree*   *Strongly agree*

14. I have forbidden foods that I don't allow myself to eat.

Strongly disagree   *Disagree*   *Neutral*   *Agree*   *Strongly agree*

15. When I'm eating, I can tell when I am getting full.

Strongly disagree   *Disagree*   *Neutral*   *Agree*   *Strongly agree*

16. I use food to help me soothe my negative emotions.

Strongly disagree   *Disagree*   *Neutral*   *Agree*   *Strongly agree*

17. I find myself eating when I am stressed out, even when I'm not physically hungry.

Strongly disagree   *Disagree*   *Neutral*   *Agree*   *Strongly agree*

18. I feel guilty if I eat a certain food that is high in calories, fat or carbohydrates.

Strongly disagree   *Disagree*   *Neutral*   *Agree*   *Strongly agree*

19. I think of a certain food as 'good' or 'bad' depending on its nutritional content.

Strongly disagree   *Disagree*   *Neutral*   *Agree*   *Strongly agree*

20. I don't trust myself around fattening foods.

Strongly disagree   *Disagree*   *Neutral*   *Agree*   *Strongly agree*

21. I don't keep certain foods in my house/apartment because I think I may lose control and eat them.

Strongly disagree   *Disagree*   *Neutral*   *Agree*   *Strongly agree*

Scoring: Positive scores (items 2, 4, 7, 8, 11, 12, 13, 15): Strongly Disagree = 1, Disagree =2, Neutral =3, Agree = 4, Strongly Agree = 5. Reverse scores (items 1, 3, 5, 6, 9, 10, 14, 16, 17, 18, 19, 20, 21): Strongly Disagree = 5, Disagree =4, Neutral =3, Agree = 2, Strongly Agree = 1.

Subscale	Unconditional Permission to Eat	Eating for Physical Rather Than Emotional Reasons	Reliance on Internal Hunger/Satiety Cues	Total score
items	1, 4, 5, 9, 14, 18, 19, 20, 21	2, 3, 6, 10, 16, 17	7, 8, 11, 12, 13, 15	1–21
Total score for these items (keeping reverse scoring code as above)				
Divide by	9	6	6	21
Final scores				

Resources

Healthy eating guidelines

The following websites give government guidelines for various countries.

Dietary Guidelines for Americans

http://www.cnpp.usda.gov/dietaryguidelines.htm

Daily Intake Guide (Australia)

http://www.mydailyintake.net/

NHS Healthy Eating (UK)

http://www.nhs.uk/livewell/healthy-eating/Pages/Healthyeating.aspx

NZ Ministry of Health Food and Nutrition Guidelines

http://www.health.govt.nz/our-work/preventative-health-wellness/nutrition/
food-and-nutrition-guidelines

South African Guidelines for Healthy Eating

ftp://ftp.fao.org/es/esn/nutrition/dietary_guidelines/zaf_eating.pdf

Marketing, advertising, consumer awareness

BBC News Health (UK)
Excellent source of regular commentary on the latest research findings. Join their RRS feed for automatic alerts.
http://www.bbc.com/news/video_and_audio/health/

Choice (Australia)
Choice offers unbiased, independent consumer information on a wide range of products and services.
http://www.choice.com.au/

Food Standards Australia New Zealand
http://www.foodstandards.gov.au

Harvard School of Public Health (USA)
Forward-thinking views on nutrition which challenge many current guidelines.
http://www.hsph.harvard.edu/

Junkbusters (Australia)
Junkbusters is a website giving Australian parents a platform to voice their concerns regarding inappropriate food advertising aimed at children.
http://junkbusters.com.au

NHS Live Well
Excellent, easy-to-read fact sheets and articles on all things health.
http://www.nhs.uk/Livewell/Goodfood/Pages/eatwell-plate.aspx

Other websites

5 A Day (NZ)
A fabulous site by New Zealand agencies on the importance of fruit and vegetables, with extensive resources for educational settings and research findings on produce and health.
http://www.5aday.co.nz

The ABC's Natural Health Guide
Reviews herbal remedies, homoeopathics and much more.
http://www.abc.net.au/health/healthyliving/naturalhealth/guide/

Brian Wansink's Mindless Eating resources
http://mindlesseating.org/

Change 4 Life (UK)
http://www.nhs.uk/change4life/Pages/change-for-life.aspx

Fat free TV (Australia)
Created by the Cancer Council, this is a fun site to check how your kids are going.
http://www.fatfreetv.com.au/daily-junk-ad-calculator

Health at Every Size
http://www.haescommunity.org/

Miracle Foods: Myths and Media, NHS (UK)
http://www.nhs.uk/news/2011/02February/Pages/miracle-foods-special-report.aspx

True Food Network (Australia)

Created by Greenpeace, the True Food Network works tirelessly to ensure safe and sustainable food.

http://www.truefood.org.au

Swap It Don't Stop It (Australia)

This website has some great online resources for healthy weight.

http://www.measureup.gov.au/internet/abhi/publishing.nsf/Content/become-a-swapper-lp

Endnotes

Introduction

1. Myers, A., 1980, 'Food accessibility and food choice', *Archives of General Psychiatry*, 37, 1133–5, cited in Shepherd and Raats (eds), *The Psychology of Food Choice*, CABI, Wallingford, UK.

Chapter 1

1. Willcox, D. Craig et al., 2009, 'The Okinawan diet: Health implications of a low-calorie, nutrient-dense, antioxidant-rich dietary pattern low in glycemic load', *Journal of the American College of Nutrition*, 28.sup4, pp. 500S–516S.

2. Sofi, F. et al., 2010, 'Accruing evidence on benefits of adherence to the Mediterranean diet on health: an updated systematic review and meta-analysis', *American Journal of Clinical Nutrition*, 92.5, pp. 1189–96.

3. Source: http://www.oecd.org/health/49716427.pdf

4. Policy Brief: Obesity Update 2012

5. http://www.cdc.gov/obesity/data/adult.html

6. Policy Brief: Obesity Update 2012

Chapter 2

1. Source: Furst, T., Connors, M., Bisogni, C., Sobal, F. and Falk, L., 1996, 'Food Choice: A conceptual model of the process', *Appetite*, 26, pp. 247–66.

2. Dressler, H. and Smith, C., 2013,'Food choice, eating behavior, and food liking differs between lean/normal and overweight/obese, low-income women', *Appetite*, vol. 26, 1 June 2013, pp. 145–52: http://www.sciencedirect.com/science/article/pii/S0195666313000342

3. Quick, V., Wall, M., Larsen, N., Haines, J. and Neumark-Sztainer, D., 2013, 'Personal, behavioral and socio-environmental predictors of overweight incidence in young adults: 10-yr longitudinal findings', *International Journal of Behavioral Nutrition and Physical Activity*, 10:37: http://www.ijbnpa.org/content/pdf/1479-5868-10-37.pdf

4. Kavanagh, A., et al., 2007, 'VicLANES: Place does matter for your health', University of Melbourne, Melbourne.

5. Chandon, P. and Wansink, B., 2012, 'Does food marketing need to make us fat? A review and solutions', *Nutrition Reviews*, 70.10, pp. 571–93.

6. Mittal, D., Stevenson, R., Oaten, M. and Miller, L., 2011 'Snacking while watching TV impairs food recall and promotes food intake on a later TV free test meal', *Applied Cognitive Psychology*, pp. 871–7.

7. Diliberti, N., Bordi, P.L., Conklin, M.T., Roe, L.S. and Rolls, B.J., 2004, 'Increased portion size leads to increased energy intake in a restaurant meal', *Obes Res*, 12(3), pp, 562–8.

Chapter 3

1. Illustration based on: http://www.ncbi.nlm.nih.gov/pubmedhealth/PMH0033701/

2. Illustration based on: Chandrashekar, J., Hoon, M.A., Ryba, N.J. and Zuker, C.S., 2006, 'The receptors and cells for mammalian taste', p. 288.

3. van Goudoever, H., Guandalini, S., Kleinman, R.E. (eds), 2011, *Early Nutrition: Impact on short- and long-term health*, Nestlé Nutrition Institute, Karger, Basel, pp. 153–68.

4. Garcia-Bailo, B., Toguri, C., Eny, K. and El-Sohemy, A., 2009, 'Review:

Genetic variation in taste and its influence on food selection', *Journal of Integrative Biology*, vol. 13, no. 1, pp. 68–80.

5.   Chale-Rush, A., Burgess, J.R. and Mattes, R.D., 2007, 'Evidence for human orosensory (taste?) sensitivity to free fatty acids', *Chem Senses*, vol. 32, pp. 423–31.

6.   Excerpt from Proietto, J., 'Do diets matter in the battle against obesity?' University of Melbourne Department of Medicine, Victoria, Australia. Nutrition Society of Australia 34th Annual Scientific Meeting Program, November 2010.

7.   Illustration based on: http://www.news-medical.net/health/What-is-the-Hypothalamus.aspx

8.   Provencher, V. et al., 2007, 'Social and behavioral short-term effects of a "health-at-every-size" approach on eating behaviors and appetite ratings', *Obesity*, 15.4, pp. 957–66.

9.   Yeomans, M and Chambers, L., 2011, 'Satiety-relevant sensory qualities enhance the satiating effect of mixed carbohydrate-protein preloads', *American Journal of Clinical Nutrition*, 94, pp. 1410–7.

10.   ibid.

Chapter 4

1.   Hendy, H.M. and Raudenbush, B., 2000, 'Effectiveness of teacher modeling to encourage food acceptance in preschool children', *Appetite*, 34.1, pp. 61–76.

2.   Illustration based on: Shepherd, R. and Raats, M., 2006, *The Psychology of Food Choice*, CABI, Wallingford, UK, p. 97.

Chapter 5

1.   Selk, J., 'Habit formation: The 21-day myth', *Forbes*, 15 April 2013:

http://www.forbes.com/sites/jasonselk/2013/04/15/habit-formation-the-21-day-myth/

2. Cosgrove, F., 2007, *Coach Yourself to Wellness: Living the intentional life.*

3. Australian Psychological Society, 2000, 'Media representations and responsibilities: Psychological perspectives': www.psychology.org.au/publications/statements/media/

4. 'Good Thinking', National Psychology Week 12–18 November 2006, Health Behaviour Change survey conducted by the Australian Psychological Society.

5. Wansink, B., 2010, 'Review: From mindless eating to mindlessly eating better', *Physiology & Behavior*, vol. 100, pp. 454–63.

6. Source of table: Koster, E.P., 2007, 'Diversity in the determinants of food choice: A psychological perspective', 'Food quality and preference' (in press), pp. 1–13.

7. Dötsch, M., Busch, J., Batenburg, M., Liem, G., Tareilus, E., Mueller, R. and Meijer, G., 2009, 'Strategies to reduce sodium consumption: A food industry perspective', *Critical Reviews in Food Science and Nutrition*, 49, pp. 841–51.

8. Baumeister, R.F., Bratslavsky, E., Muraven, M. and Tice, D.M., 1998, 'Ego depletion: Is the active self a limited resource?', *Journal of Personality and Social Psychology*, vol. 74(5), pp. 1252–65.

Chapter 6

1. Martin, F.J., Antille, N., Rezzi, S. and Kochhar, S., 2012, 'Everyday eating experiences of chocolate and non-chocolate snacks impact postprandial anxiety, energy and emotional states', *Nutrients*, vol. 4, pp. 554–67.

2. van Strien, T. et al., 2012, 'Moderation of distress-induced eating by emotional eating scores', *Appetite*, 58.1, pp. 277–84.

3. Elfhaga, K. and Moreyb, L., 2008, 'Personality traits and eating behavior in the obese: Poor self-control in emotional and external eating but personality assets in restrained eating', *Eating Beh*, vol. 9, pp. 285–93.

4. Munro, I.A. et al., 2011, 'Using personality as a predictor of diet induced weight loss and weight management', *International Journal of Behavioral Nutrition and Physical Activity*, 8.1, pp. 1–9.

5. Temple, J.L. et al., 2008, 'Overweight children find food more reinforcing and consume more energy than do nonoverweight children', *American Journal of Clinical Nutrition*, 87.5, pp. 1121–7.

6. Rotter, J.B., 1966, 'Generalized expectancies of internal versus external control of reinforcements', *Psychological Monographs*, 80, p. 609.

7. Gale, C.R., Batty, G.D. and Deary, I.J., 2008, 'Locus of control at age 10 years and health outcomes and behaviors at age 30 years: The 1970 British cohort study', *Psychosomatic Medicine*, 70, pp. 397–403.

Chapter 7

1. Source: Strategic Business Insights.

2. Lang, T. and Millstone, E. (eds), 2002, *The Atlas of Food*, Earthscan Books, cited in Dalmeny, K., Hanna, E. and Lobstein, T., 2003 'Broadcasting bad health', International Association of Consumer Food Organizations.

3. Consumers International, www.consumersinternational.org.

4. http://www.weeklytimesnow.com.au/article/2010/08/02/214531_business-news.html

5. Conner, M. and Armitage, C., 2002, *The Social Psychology of Food*, Open University Press, Maidenhead, UK.

6. Robinson, T.N. et al., 2007, 'Effects of fast food branding on young children's taste preferences', *Archives of Pediatrics & Adolescent Medicine*, 161.8, pp. 792–7.

7. Harris, J.L., Bargh, J.A. and Brownell, K.D., 2009, 'Priming effects of television food advertising on eating behavior', *Health Psychology*, vol. 28, no. 4, pp. 404–13.

8. Jones, S., Andrews, K., Tapsell, L., Williams, P. and McVie, D., 2008, 'The extent and nature of "health messages" in magazine food advertising in Australia', *Asia Pacific Journal of Clinical Nutrition*, vol. 17 (2), pp. 317–24.

9. Mikkelsen, L., Merlo, C., Lee, V. and Chao, C., 2007 '*Where's the fruit?: Fruit content of the most highly-advertised children's food and beverages*', Prevention Institute.

10. http://www.fastfoodmarketing.org/fast_food_facts_in_brief.aspx

11. ibid.

Chapter 8

1. European Prospective Investigation into Cancer and Nutrition, 2009.

2. http://www.bda.uk.com/foodfacts/TransFats.pdf

3. Bialkova, S. and van Trijp, H., 'What determines consumer attention to nutrition labels?', *Food Quality and Preference*, vol. 21, issue 8, December 2010, pp. 1042–51.

4. Williams, P., 2005, 'Consumer understanding and use of health claims for foods', *Nutrition Reviews*, vol. 63(7), pp. 256–64.

5. Australian Division of World Action on Salt and Health (AWASH), 2007, 'Survey of Australian consumer awareness and practices relating to salt: report', George Institute for International Health, Australia.

Appendix 1

1. Van Strien et al., (1986). The Dutch Eating Behaviour Questionnaire (DEBQ) for assessment of restrained, emotional and external eating behaviour, *International Journal of Eating Disorders*, 5(2), pp. 295–315.

Appendix 2

1. Tylka, T. L. (2006). Development and psychometric evaluation of a measure of intuitive eating, *Journal of Counseling Psychology*, 53(2), pp. 226–240.

Bibliography

Arimond, M. and Ruel, M., 2004 'Dietary diversity is associated with child nutritional status: Evidence from 11 demographic health surveys', *Journal of Nutrition*, 134, pp. 2579–85.

Australian Bureau of Statistics, 2002, 'National Health Survey — Summary of results, Canberra.

Australian Division of World Action on Salt and Health (AWASH), 2008, 'Drop the Salt! Food industry strategy', draft for consultation.

—— 2010, 'Response to FSANZ media release on Australian salt intakes', The George Institute for International Health, Australia.

Australian Government, Department of Agriculture, Fisheries and Forestry, 2006, Australian Food Statistics, Food and Agriculture Division, Canberra.

—— Department of Health and Aging, 2008, Australian Food and Grocery Council and Australian Government Department of Agriculture, Fisheries and Forestry, '2007 Australian National Children's Nutrition and Physical Activity Survey'.

—— Australian Communications and Media Authority, 2007, 'Television advertising to children: A review of contemporary research on the influence of television advertising directed to children', Prepared for ACMA by Dr Jeffrey E. Brand.

Baumeister, R.F., Bratslavsky, E., Muraven, M. and Tice, D.M., 1998, 'Ego depletion: Is the active self a limited resource?' *Journal of Personality and Social Psychology*, 74(5), pp. 1252–65.

Bargh, J.A., Chen, M. and Burrows, L., 1996, 'Automaticity of social behavior: Direct effects of trait construct and stereotype-activation on action', *Journal of Personality and Social Psychology*, 71(2), pp. 230–44.

Barthomeuf, L., Rousset, S. and Droit-Volet, S., 2009, 'Emotion and food: Do the emotions expressed on other people's faces affect the desire to eat liked and disliked food products?' *Appetite*, 52, pp. 27–33.

Beard, T., Woodward, D., Ball, P., Hornsby, H., von Witt, R. and Dwyer, T., 1997, 'The Hobart Salt Study 1995: Few meet national sodium intake target', *Medical Journal of Australia*, 166, p. 404.

Bell, R. and Pliner, P., 2003, 'Time to eat: The relationship between the number of people eating and meal duration in three lunch settings', *Appetite*, 41, pp. 215–18.

Birch, L., McPhee, L., Shoba, B., Pirok, E. and Steinberg, L., 1987, 'What kind of exposure reduces children's food neophobia? Looking vs. tasting', *Appetite*, 9(3), pp. 171–8.

Clark, J. and Berstein, I., 2006, 'Sensitization of salt appetite is associated with increased "wanting" but not "liking" of a salt reward in the sodium-deplete rat', *Behavioral Neuroscience*, February, 120(1), pp. 206–10.

Colby, S., Johnson, L., Scheett, A. and Hoverson, B., 2010, 'Nutrition marketing on food labels', *Journal of Nutrition Education and Behavior*, March–April, 42(2), pp. 92–8.

Cooke, L., Carnell, S. and Wardle, J., 2006, 'Food neophobia and mealtime food consumption in 4–5 year old children', *International Journal of Behavioral Nutrition and Physical Activity*, 3, p. 14.

Cooke, L., Wardle, J., Gibson, E., Sapochnik, M., Sheiham, A. and Lawson, M., 2003, 'Demographic, familial and trait predictors of fruit and vegetable consumption by pre-school children', *Public Health Nutrition*, 7(2), pp. 295–302.

Cooke, L., Wardle, J. and Gibson, E., 2003, 'Relationship between parental report of food neophobia and everyday food consumption in 2–6 year old children', *Appetite*, 41, pp. 205–6.

Contreras, R., Kosten, T. and Frank, M., 1984, 'Activity in salt taste fibers: Peripheral mechanism for mediating changes in salt intake', *Chemical Senses*, 8, pp. 275–88.

Cowburn, G. and Stockley, L., 2004, 'Consumer understanding and use of nutrition labelling: A systematic review', *Public Health Nutrition*, 8(1), pp. 21–8.

Carruth, B. and Skinner, J., 2000, 'Revisiting the picky eater phenomenon: Neophobic behaviours in young children', *Journal of the American College of Nutrition*, 19, no. 6, pp. 771–80.

Delva, J., O'Malley, P. and Johnston, L., 2007, 'Availability of more-healthy and less-healthy food choices in American schools: A national study of grade, racial/ethnic, and socioeconomic differences', *American Journal of Preventive Medicine*, Oct, 33(4 suppl), pp. S226–39.

Edwards, J. and Meiselman, H., 2005, 'The influence of positive and negative cues on restaurant choice and food acceptance', *International Journal of Contemporary Hospitality Management*, 17, pp. 332–44.

Edwards, J., Meiselman, H., Edwards, A. and Lesher, L., 2003, 'The influence of eating location on the acceptability of identically prepared foods', *Food Quality and Preference*, 14, pp. 647–52.

Ekstein, S., Laniado, D. and Glick, B., 2010, 'Does picky eating affect weight-for-length measurements in young children?' *Clinical Pediatrics*, vol. 49, issue 3, pp. 217–20.

Falciglia, G., Couch, S., Gribble, L., Pabst, S. and Frank, R., 2000, 'Food neophobia in childhood affects dietary variety', *Journal of the American Dietetic Association*, 100(12), pp. 1474–81.

Finlayson, G., King, N. and Blundell, J., 2007, 'Is it possible to dissociate "liking" and "wanting" for foods in humans? A novel experimental procedure', *Physiology and Behavior*, 30 January, 90(1), pp. 36–42.

Flight, I., Leppard, P. and Cox, D., 2003, 'Food neophobia and associations with cultural diversity and socio-economic status amongst rural and urban Australian adolescents', *Appetite*, 41, pp. 51–9.

Forouhi, N. et al., 2009, 'Dietary fat intake and subsequent weight change in adults: Results from the European Prospective Investigation into Cancer and Nutrition cohorts 1–3', *American Journal of Clinicial Nutrition*, 90, pp. 1632–41.

Friese, M., Hofmann, W. and Wanke, M., 2008, 'When impulses take over: Moderated predictive validity of explicit and implicit attitude measures in predicting food choice and consumption behaviour', *British Journal of Social Psychology*, 47, pp. 397–419.

Furst, T., Connors, M., Bisogni, C., Sobal, F. and Falk, L., 1996, 'Food choice: A conceptual model of the process', *Appetite*, 26, pp. 247–66.

Galloway, A., Lee, Y. and Birch, L., 2003, 'Predictors and consequences of food neophobia and pickiness in young girls', *Journal of the American Dietetic Association*, June, 103(6), pp. 692–8.

Ganchrow, J. and Mennella, J., 2003, 'The ontogeny of human flavour perception' in *Handbook of Olfaction and Gustation*, 2nd ed., Marcel Dekker Inc., New York, pp. 823–846.

Gilbey, A. and Fifield, S., 2006, 'Nutritional information about sodium: Is it worth its salt?', *New Zealand Medical Journal*, 119(1232), pp. U1937.

Grimes, C., Riddell, L. and Nowson, C., 2009, 'Consumer knowledge and attitudes to salt intake and labelled salt information', *Appetite*, October, 53(2), pp. 189–94.

Guardia, M., Guerrero, L., Gelabert, J., Gou, P. and Arnau, J., 2006, 'Consumer attitude towards sodium reduction in meat products and acceptability of fermented sausages with reduced sodium content', *Meat Science*, 73, pp. 484–90.

Harris, L., Bargh, J. and Brownell, K., 2009, 'Priming effects of television food advertising on eating behavior', *Health Psychology*, July, 28(4) pp. 404–13, doi:10.1037/a0014399.

Hayes, J., Sullivan, B. and Duffy, V., 2010, 'Explaining variability in sodium intake thorough oral sensory phenotype, salt sensation and liking', *Physiology and Behavior*, 16 June, 100(4), pp. 369–380.

Hays, N. and Roberts, S., 2008, 'Aspects of eating behaviors "disinhibition" and "restraint" are related to weight gain and BMI in women', *Obesity* (Silver Spring), January, 16(1), pp. 52–8.

Henney, J., Taylor, C. and Boon, C. (eds), 2010, *Strategies to reduce sodium intake in the United States*, National Academies Press, Washington.

International Fruit and Vegetable Alliance, 2006, 'Fruit, vegetable and health: A scientific overview', Canada. Re-printed in New Zealand by United Fresh.

Johnson, R. et al., 2009, 'Dietary sugars intake and cardiovascular health: A scientific statement from the American Heart Association', 120, pp. 1011–20.

Jones, S., Andrews, K., Tapsell, L., Williams, P. and McVie, D., 2008, 'The extent and nature of "health messages" in magazine food advertising in Australia', *Asia Pacific Journal of Clinical Nutrition*, 17(2), pp. 317–24.

Kramer, F., Lesher, L. and Meiselman, H., 1992, 'Monotony and choice: Repeated servings of the same item to soldiers under field conditions', *Appetite*, 36, pp. 239–40.

Kuchler, F. and Lin, B., 2002, 'The influence of individual choices and attitudes on adiposity', *International Journal of Obesity and Related Metabolic Disorders*, July, 26(7), pp. 1017–22.

Leshem, M., 2009, 'The excess salt appetite of humans is not due to sodium loss in adulthood', *Physiology and Behavior*, 7 September, 98(3), pp. 331–7.

Loewen, R. and Pliner, P., 2000, 'The food situations questionnaire: A measure of children's willingness to try novel foods in stimulating and non-stimulating situations', *Appetite*, December, 35(3), pp. 329–50.

Mattes, R., 1997, 'The taste for salt in humans', *American Journal of Clinical Nutrition*, 65(suppl), pp. 692S–7S.

Meiselman, H., Hedderley, D., Staddon, S., Pierson, B. and Symonds, C., 1994, 'Effect of effort on meal selection and meal acceptability in a student cafeteria', *Appetite*, 23, pp. 43–55.

Mennella, J., Jagnow, C. and Beauchamp, G., 2001, 'Prenatal and postnatal flavor learning by human infants', *Pediatrics*, June, 107(6), p. E88.

Mhurchu, C. and Gorton, D., 2007, 'Nutrition labels and claims in New Zealand and Australia: A review of use and understanding', *Australian and New Zealand Journal of Public Health*, 31(2), pp. 105–112.

Miller, M. and Pollard, C., 2005, 'Health working with industry to promote fruit and vegetables: A case study of the Western Australian Fruit and Vegetable Campaign with reflection on effectiveness of inter-sectoral action', *Australian and New Zealand Journal of Public Health*, April, 29(2), pp. 176–82.

Monneuse, M. et al., 2008, 'Taste acuity of obese adolescents and changes in food neophobia and food preferences during a weight reduction session', *Appetite*, 50, 2–3, pp. 302–7.

National Salt Initiative, implementing the EU Framework for salt reduction initiatives, June 2009.

National Health and Medical Research Council (NHMRC), 2003, *Dietary Guidelines for Children and Adolescents in Australia incorporating the Infant Feeding Guidelines for Health Workers*.

Northstone, K., Emmett, P., Nethersole, F. and the ALSPAC team, 2001, 'The effect of age of introduction to lumpy solids on foods eaten and reported feeding difficulties at 6 and 15 months', *Journal of Human Nutrition and Dietetics*, 14, pp. 43–54.

Ouwehand, C. and Papies, E., 2010, 'Eat it or beat it: The differential effects of food temptations on overweight and normal-weight restrained eaters', *Appetite*, 55, pp. 56–60.

Papies, E., Stroebe, W. and Aarts, H., 2008, 'The allure of forbidden food: On the role of attention in self-regulation', *Journal of Experimental Social Psychology*, 44, pp. 1283–92.

Pliner, P. and Hobden, K., 1992, 'Development of a scale to measure the trait of food neophobia in humans', *Appetite*, 19, pp. 105–20.

Pulos, E. and Leng, K., 2010, 'Evaluation of a voluntary menu-labeling program in full-service restaurants', *American Journal of Public Health*, June, 100(6), pp. 1035–9.

Remick, A., Polivy, J. and Pliner, P., 2009, 'Internal and external moderators of the effect of variety on food intake', *Psychological Bulletin*, American Psychological Association, vol. 135, no. 3, pp. 434–51

Roberto, C.A., Larsen, P.D., Agnew, H., Baik, J. and Brownell, K.D., 2010, 'Evaluating the impact of menu labeling on food choices and intake', *American Journal of Public Health*, February, 100(2), pp. 312–8.

Russel, C. and Worsley, A., 2008, 'A population-based study of preschoolers' food neophobia and its associations with food preferences', *Journal of Nutrition Education and Behavior*, 40(1), pp. 11–19.

Salbe, A., DelParigi, A., Pratley, R., Drewnowski, A. and Tataranni, P., 2004, 'Taste preferences and body weight changes in an obesity-prone population', *American Journal of Clinical Nutrition*, March, vol. 79, no. 3, pp. 372–8.

Schwartz, C., Issanchou, S. and Nicklaus, S., 2009, 'Developmental changes in the acceptance of the five basic tastes in the first year of life', *British Journal of Nutrition*, November, 102(9), pp. 1375–85.

Segovia, G., Hutchinson, I., Laing, D. and Jinks, A., 2002, 'A quantitative study of fungi form papillae and taste pore density in adults and children', *Developmental Brain Research*, 138, pp. 135–146.

Shepherd, R. and Farleigh, C., 1986, 'Preferences, attitudes and personality as determinants of salt intake', *Human Nutrition: Applied Nutrition*, June, 40(3), pp. 195–208.

Stroebe, W., Mensink Henk, W., Henk Schut, A. and Kruglanski, A., 2007, 'Why dieters fail: Testing the goal conflict model of eating', *Journal of Experimental Social Psychology*, 44, 1, p. 26.

Subar, A., Krebs-Smith, S., Cook, A. and Kahle, L., 1998, 'What kind of exposure reduces children's food neophobia?' *Journal of the American Dietetic Association*, 98(5), pp. 537–47.

Terracciano, A. et al., 2009, 'Facets of personality linked to underweight and overweight', *Psychosomatic Medicine*, July, 71(6), pp. 682–9.

Turrell, G., Blakely, T., Patterson, C. and Oldenburg, B., 2004, 'A multilevel analysis of socioeconomic (small area) differences in household food purchasing behaviour', *Journal of Epidemiology and Community Health*, March, 58(3), pp. 208–15.

Van der Veen, J., De Graaf, C., Van Dis, S. and Staveren, W., 1999, 'Determinants of salt use in cooked meals in the Netherlands: Attitudes and practices of food preparers', *European Journal of Clinical Nutrition*, 53, pp. 288–394.

Wansink, B., van Ittersum, K. and Painter, J., 2005, 'How descriptive food names bias sensory perceptions in restaurants', *Food Quality and Preference*, 16, pp. 393–100.

Wardle, J. and Cooke, L., 2008, 'Genetic and environmental determinants of children's food preferences', *British Journal of Nutrition*, 99(1), pp. 15–21.

Wardle, J. et al., 2003, 'Increasing children's acceptance of vegetables: A randomized trial of parent-led exposure', *Appetitie*, 40, 2, pp. 155–62.

Webster, J., Dunford, E. and Neal, B., 2009, 'A systematic survey of the sodium contents of processed foods', *American Journal of Clinical Nutrition*, December, p. 10.

World Cancer Research Fund/American Institute for Cancer Research, 2007, *Food, Nutrition, Physical Activity, and the Prevention of Cancer: A global perspective*, AICR Washington DC.

World Health Organization, 2002, 'Diet, physical activity and health — a global response', (Department of NCDs), December.

—— 2002, 'World Health Report 2002: Reducing risks, promoting healthy life', Geneva.

—— 2007, '2008–2013 Action Plan for the Global Strategy for the Prevention and Control of Noncommunicable Diseases'.

—— 2005, 'Participants at the 6th Global Conference on Health Promotion. The Bangkok Charter for health promotion in a globalized world', Geneva.

Williams, K., Riegel, K. and Kerwin, M., 2009, 'Feeding disorder of infancy or early childhood: How often is it seen in feeding programs?', *Children's Health Care*, 38, pp. 123–36.

Worsley, A., 2000, 'Food and consumers: Where are we heading?', *Asia Pacific Journal of Clinical Nutrition*, 9(suppl.), pp. S103–7.

—— 2002, 'Nutrition knowledge and food consumption: Can nutrition knowledge change food behaviour?', *Asia Pacific Journal of Clinical Nutrition*, 11(suppl.), pp. S579–85.

Index

A
Achievers *160–1*
adolescents *see* teenagers
advertising
  effect on eating 166–7
  food 164
  goals of 163–4
  in magazines 167
  pay attention to 165
  using personalities 177
agreeableness (Big 5 trait) 141
appetite 54
aromas, in food context 27
artificial sweeteners 47, 97
Australia, obesity levels 12
Australian Psychological Society (APS)
  study
    change of eating habits 111
    obese people 138–9
automatic behaviour
  eating as 124
  effort to control 131–2
  strength of 122–4
  understanding 121–2

B
behavioural change
  adjustments chart 117
  barriers to 103
  factors for 145
  maintaining 111
Believers *160–1*
benzaldehyde, flavour of 97
Big 5 Model personality traits 141–2
bitter taste 40, *43*, 45, 48
body cues
  becoming familiar with 76
  importance of 71–9
  rating chart *78*
body wisdom 55
brain, hunger control 57–9
branding 165–6
bread, sodium/salt levels 176

C
calories, counting 3
carbohydrates 170–1
changes, pointers for making 180–2
children
  eating cues 55
  fussy eaters 46
  peer influence 95
  salty food 67
  tastebuds 41
children's food, US packaging 167
chocolate
  impulse purchase 32
  lower anxiety 134
cholecystokinin (CCK) hormone 56
cholesterol 8, 172
circumvallate papillae 42, *43*, 51
classical conditioning 88–90, *99*
coffee
  post-ingestive effects of 98–9
  reducing intake 115–6
commitment, eating habits 143
conscientiousness (Big 5 trait) 141
  restrained eaters 143
consumer segments 156, *157*, *158*,
  160–1, 162
Cosgrove, Fiona 103, 105–6
cravings 60–1
cruciferous vegetables 8

D
decision-making styles 125–6
depolarisation 48–9
diet soda, weight gain link 80
dietary fibre 8
dieting
  current paradigm 72–3
  reality about 128–9
diets
  basic principles 7–10
  failure of 132
  for longevity 10–1
direct advertising 164
dog conditioning 88–9

E

eating
   automatic behaviour 124
   conscious 16
   controlling the urge 126
   dynamic 9
   and habits 119–21
   pleasure of 59–60
eating habits
   changing 104–7, 113–4, 114, 115
   formation process 102–4
   hardest to change 118–9
   ingrained 101–2
   learning processes 95, 96
   life stages 19
   obstacles to formation 103
   re-evaluating 17–8
   reshaping 72–4, 98
   social influences 62–4
   'unlearning' 119
   see also food choices
emotional eating 135–40
endorsements
   famous people 95
   on food products 177
Experiencers 158, *160–1*
external influences
   food choices 61–2
   food intake *39*
extraversion (Big 5 trait) 141

F

Facebook ads, fast food outlets 167
fat taste perception 50–1
fats
   'less desirable' 51, 52
   tips to consider 172–3
Fatty Acid Transporter (FAT) 51
fatty acids 50–1
fatty foods, preference for 69
fear of new food 99–100
fibre, dietary 8
filiform papillae *43*
flavour, infants' preferences 97
flavour-consequence learning (FCL)
   97–8

foetuses, taste and smell 44, 65–6
foliate papillae 42, *43*, 51
food
   access to 24–5
   approach to 94
   fear of new food 99–100
   post-ingestive effects of 98–9
   view of 6
food characteristics, influence on satiety
   83
food choice models, importance of
   14–5
food choices
   classical conditioning 89
   contextual factors 26–9
   influences over 20, 34–5, 61–2,
      135–40
   personal factors 20, 23–4
   social framework 25–6
   socio-economic status 24–6
   strategies 34–5
   tips for 177–8
   triggers for bad choices 120–1
   US weight study 23
   see also eating habits
food context
   change strategy 30–1
   increased consumption 26–9
food groups, variety within 7–8
food intake
   change strategy 30–1
   factors affecting 82–3
   ignoring body cues 55
   influencing factors 39
   mindless eating 28
   regulating 53–4, 56–7
food labelling 169, 173–4
food psychology, understanding 2–4
food shopping script 36
fullness *see* satiety
fungiform papillae 42, *43*, 49
Furst Model of Food Choice 14, 16–7,
   18
fussy eaters 44, 46, 64

G
genes, taste control 48
ghrelin, hunger stimulant 56
glucose transporters 46
goals
    medium-term 110
    self-monitoring 109
    setting 105, 108, 180
    SMART model 106–7
'goldfish', mind map 87

H
Health at Every Size (HAES) approach
    73, 132–3
health claims, food products 175–6
'hedonic hunger' 71
hunger
    bad food choices 80
    brain control function 57–9
    create own scale 77
    explained 54
    fatty foods 69–70
    feeling of 76
    levels of 75
    psychological 71
hypothalamus
    response to hunger 57–8
    structure 58
    weight control role 56

I
ice-cream as a reward 92–3
ideals
    about weight 23
    food-related 21–2
    personal 20
imitation, learning by 94–5
impulsivity, BMI link 142
inhibition eating 98
Innovators 160–1
instrumental conditioning 90–1
internal factors
    affecting taste 39–45, 48–61
    food intake 39
Intuitive Eating Scale 189–92

L
learning processes
    classical conditioning 88–90, 99
    food habits 95, 96
    imitation 94–5
    instrumental conditioning 90–1
    memory system 87
lighting, in food context 27
liking vs wanting 64–5
liquid 'foods' 80–1
Locus of Control (LOC)
    emotional response to outcomes 150,
    151
    internal LOC 151–2
    internal/external examples 147–50
    recognising statements 153–4
    relevance 146
logos on food products 177
longevity, diets for 10–1
low-fat products 171, 173

M
Makers 160–1
market segments see consumer segments
marketing
    advertising costs 159
    the four Ps 163
    non-commercial 156
    psychographic segmentation 156–8
McDonald's
    advertising budget 167
    product launch 159
memory system 87
mindful eating 16
mindless eating, food intake 28
monoamine neurotransmitters 83
monosodium glutamate 50
motivation, and weight control 144–52
motivators vs locus of control 146
music, in food context 27, 63

N
negative reinforcement 91, 92
neuroticism (Big 5 trait) 141, 143
neurotransmitters, influence on mood
    83

non-nutritive sweeteners 47, 97
nutrition 5–6
nutrition panels 168–73
nutritional needs, individual 9–10

O

obesity
    adult OECD rates 12–3, *12*
    APS study results 138–9
    developing countries 11
    Okinawa, Japan, diet 10–1
    100g column, nutrition panels 169
openness (Big 5 trait) 141
operant psychology 90–1

P

packaging
    information on 174
    US children's food 167
palatability 60, 70–1
papillae
    'supertasters' 66
    types 42
parasympathetic nervous system 135
Pavlov, Ivan 88–9
peer influence 95
'per serve' column, nutrition panels
    169–70
peripheral advertising 164
personal systems, eating habits 32
personality
    effect on eating 142–4
    and weight control 140–4
personality profiling 141–2
physical activity 139
plant foods, for longevity 10–1
polyunsaturated fats, cholesterol 8
portion sizes, reducing 10, 28, 29, 105,
    113–4
positive punishers 91
pre-absorptive metabolic phase of
    digestion 47
processed foods, dietary salt 176
protein, stimulates satiety 79, 82
punishers, positive and negative 91–3

Q

questionnaires
    Dutch Eating Behaviour 183–8
    Intuitive Eating Scale 189–92
    rating areas 137

R

rating scales 105
'rebound hunger' 80
receptors, fatty acid 50–1
repetition, effect of 126
resistance levels, mode of learning *118*
resources, access to food 24–5
restrained eaters 128–9, 143
restraint
    eating habits 121, 143
    energy used by 130–2
rewards
    appropriate *93*
    intrinsic/extrinsic 146
    understanding impact 91–4

S

salt
    food labelling 175–6
    reducing intake 68, 84
salty taste
    change strategies 119
    perception process 49
    preference for 66–7
    tastebud zone *43*
Sardinia, Italy, diet 11
satiation, explained 54
satiety
    create own scale 77
    different food types 79
    expectation of 81–3
    feeling of 76
    levels of 75
    psychology of 82–3
    sensory-specific (SSS) 81–3
saturated fatty acids
    cholesterol 8
    knowledge update 51–2
savoury taste 40, 45, 50, 82
self-monitoring

body cues 77, 79
goals 109
rating chart *78*
successful change 105–6
Selk, Jason 102–3
sensory-specific satiety (SSS) 81–3
serotonin 83
shelf location 34
shopping habits 34–5, 36–7
'silent teacher modelling' 94–5
simple sugars 170
Skinner, B.J. 90
SMART goals 106–7
social facilitation, influence on eating 62–4
social learning theory 94–5
socio-economic status, food choices 24–6
sodium, food labelling 175–6
sour taste 40, *43*, 48–9
stress
    effect on eating 135, 137–40
    life stage influences 19
Strivers *160–1*
Stroop Effect 122–4, *123*
success, tips to improve 111–2
sugars 97, 170
supplements 9
Survivors 158, *160–1*
sweet taste 40, *43*, 45, 46, 82
sweet tooth 65

T
taste physiology 40, 53
taste preferences 65–6, 84
taste sensations
    development 45–51
    early start 44
    timeline for 97
taste sensitivity 44
tastebuds
    location and function 41, *42*
    tongue receptors *43*
tastes, repeated exposure 99–100
teenagers
    eating habits 19

peer pressure 62
    weight control behaviours 24
Thinkers *160–1*
trans fats, food labelling 171–2
tryptophan 83–4
TV, eating in front of 28

U
umami taste 40, 45, 50, 82
unprocessed food 9
US food labelling 169

V
VALS framework 156, *157*, 158
value negotiations 32, 33
variety
    within food groups 7–8
    of foods 7, 126
vegetarians, social framework 26
VicLANES study 24–5
vision
    overall 105–6
    setting yours 108

W
wanting vs liking 64–5
websites, food information related 193–6
weight control
    and motivation 144–52
    non-diet perspective 132
    and personality 140–4
weight gain
    diet soda link 80
    non-nutritive sweeteners 47
weight regain 56
weight-loss diet, difficulty with 85
weight-loss industry 55
whole ingredients 9